FIREFIGHTER NUTRITION PLAN

INTRODUCTION

Firefighting jobs are tough to find nowadays. The requirements and criteria determined by the fire departments have grown lately as a result of requirement on program. This is not to say you don't have a prospect of being a firefighter. There are several distinct techniques to get into this incredible livelihood; you merely need to maintain an open mind.

Working as a firefighter you have to experience a number of tasks. You have the chance to concentrate in a great deal of areas. You are able to go down the route of being a paramedic, an emergency medical technician, volunteer firefighter, fire inspector, and also a lot more. So it isn't to say your choices simply revolve around turning into a fulltime firefighter.

You may not understand your market until you really start operating in the surroundings. Some people's perceptions shift once confronted with the daily activities of a project. The very best thing is that if you have a fire for this particular profession then there's something inside which will agree with your qualities and abilities!

There's a very long road to travel before you step foot onto a fire truck or truck. Listed below are a couple of the procedures you'll have to undergo when searching for firefighting jobs:

Research - get to know different kinds of jobs out there. Look into every business in detail and also become knowledgeable about the sort of work involved and the kind of cases you might be attending. Research the department you want to use to. This is essential since it will provide you an awareness of the region and when there'll be a number of firefighting tasks out there. Find out more about the firefighter salary that this will provide you a good notion about what to anticipate. Another excellent suggestion for when you're in the study phase of your trip is to speak to your regional fire department and ask for a day's job expertise. Most fire homes are delighted to match and forthcoming firefighters and will answer any queries or questions you might have. Most importantly, however, you'll be able to feel that the air and see for your self exactly what lays before you!

Education - even though a degree isn't essential to connect with the fire department, there are a number of things you can do this will improve your probability of being hired. There are classes offered in a number of schools around the globe offering diplomas, certifications and high credentials in emt (emergency medical technician), fire safety, fire science, hazardous materials, paramedic instruction, emergency medical dispatcher, etc., etc.. These may be short lessons and can enhance your chances by demonstrating the interviewers that you get a real interest in your job.

Physical training - this goes without saying that a solid physical health is paramount to the profession. It's not a desk job which is made up of sitting day. You'll be always active and need to get ready for any result when arriving at a crisis scenario. You don't understand what you may face on the opposite side be ready for instance; to take a 15 stone guy down 3 flights of stairs all on your own personal, in extreme heat and inadequate visibility! This isn't over exaggerating, it's a really realistic situation and trust me that there are far more challenging tasks ahead. Be under no illusion, so you'll be pushed to your limits, so be ready, you can begin now with a nutritious diet program and establishing your physical power!

The written exam - this may seem daunting for any individual. Everybody's capabilities differ in regards to examinations. The strain of this evaluation, their personal ability to comprehend questions, their capacity to keep information. What i wish to get across is it is not the end of the street should you're feeling this isn't your very best strength. You've got the chance of a meeting with a board to acquire across your want for your occupation and showcase your abilities and character. But it's necessary to get any knowledge, so when this isn't your forte nevertheless give it all and study just as far as possible. Give it your very best shot! Leave yourself be no uncertainty in your head that you did whatever you can.

The interview - today is your opportunity to shine. You've been through the breed of the written examination, you've researched and trained firefighting tasks completely, today show them exactly what you've . Be yourself, don't attempt and lie or cover up that you have, it works. People today employ people, not a manufactured character or what's on paper. Be succinct, enthused, and concentrated. Bear in mind the folks sitting on the board aren't there to find fault with you, they would like you to be successful!

Let the games begin - should you arrive at the point and have been effective in the interview period then now is whenever the exciting times begin! You may move recruit (or newcomer) training. The travel until today has been lengthy but you must stay focused and make certain you surpass all expectations when searching for firefighting tasks. To be a firefighter is among the hardest processes to survive. You'll be trained , emotionally and strategically. You may come from the and walk in the fire house as a firefighter!

The following chapter within this travel takes on a lot of different facets! It's a book alone. So begin now. Follow your fantasy and together with the step-by-step instructions above and you can't go much wrong! There's also a great deal of information available on the background of firefighting and global firefighting so utilize the world wide web to your benefit!

Water. It is vital to cell function, everyday life and optimum athletic performance. In this day of day flood us with pop, fruit beverages and sugar packed athletic beverages, it can be quite tough to make the ideal choice in regards to your hydration. Within the following guide, i will try to set you on the ideal route to correct hydration.

So just how much water do you consume daily? Can you subscribe to this older 8 glasses of water per day? Based on a 2002 study published in the American journal of physiology that the older 8 glasses of water every day is in reality, an'old fashioned' thing. According to the researcher, heinz valtin," there's absolutely not any reason a healthier adult living in a temperate climate not participated in physical activity must have a great deal of plain water. However, since someone who participates in massive quantities of rigorous physical action, and of course my occupation which ends in sweating buckets in my personal bunker-gear for the easiest of calls, you will find people that really demand more hydration compared to the typical human.

High-intensity athletes should really sign up for the older 8 glasses per day - and then some!

The reality is that a lot people walk around daily in a dried state and we do not even understand it. The body consists of approximately 60 percent water, and the mind can have up to 70 percent. There are 3 means that the body loses water, faces, and insensible loses. Insensible water loss happens in 2 ways: via exhalation of water vapor from the lungs and through sweat (sweat). Consequently, we're losing water all of the time. If we work deeply or battle a fire, the weight reduction is much greater.

The body is able to lose 1-2 gallons of fluid each hour when working superbly. Some early signs of dehydration may include:

- dry, tacky mouth

- feeling lethargic

- headache

- dizziness/lightheadedness

When not addressed, it is possible to achieve moderate to severe dehydration. This may result in heat exhaustion or heatstroke. Heatstroke is a life threatening illness that has to be fixed immediately. Your very best choice is to just prevent this dilemma by staying hydrated! When at the office i go out of the way to drink a huge glass of water through-out daily. If you get called out to a fire when you're already thirsty (like a firefighter i will attest to the firsthand!) , this may be especially harmful and also perform it's way in being a life-threatening error.

You will find numerous approaches that you are

able to figure out the quantity of water that you want to consume to stay hydrated if you're in to high-intensity and hard workouts. The formulation i register to is to drink half your body weight in oz of plain water. I consider 170lb, so i want to consume 85oz of water each day simply to stay hydrated. Today you might be thinking"wow, that's a good deal of plain water!!" and you are right, it's! It may be a struggle to consume this much water daily. You've got to be meticulous and have a strategy in place. As soon as i started badly paying attention for my own water consumption, i'd use a 1 liter nalgene water bottle. 1 liter of fluid is equivalent to 33.8 oz of water that is significantly less than half my required daily consumption of plain water. An obstacle i had to face was the understanding that my everyday water intake worked out to about 2.5 of these bottles each day! This might seem insignificant, but that notion alone actually bothered me! To fix the matter, i discovered myself a 16 oz nalgene bottle. I find it a whole lot simpler to consume the required quantity of water utilizing a bigger container. It was a psychological thing for me personally, but that is what worked!

It is important not to forget that not all of the water that your body needs on a daily basis needs to be obtained from a jar or you obtain water in the food that you consume. It might be easy to overdo it pay attention to the food that you eat too through-out daily. Almost 20 percent of the ordinary adult's water consumption comes out of their meals. For an notion of just how much water that you eat from the meals, keep a food journal (that will help you pinpoint exactly what your diet is similar to at the first position) and compute it to get a rough thought (only google'food water material' to get a large number of sites offering graphs for this advice).

Firefighter diet

Firefighting is a demanding job that will need 6,000 calories (kilocalories) daily. Firefighters who don't eat sufficient calories will get exhausted and eliminate body fat and muscle. Consuming a lot of calories within the months and weeks of a busy fire season may impair immune function and result in illness. This really isn't the opportunity to drop weight. Firefighters should test their weight every two weeks to track their energy equilibrium. The very best time to contemplate is at the morning prior to breakfast (however after menopause). Energy (calories) stems from fat, carbohydrate, and protein.)

Carbohydrate

Carbohydrate is converted into sugar and stored in muscle and liver as glycogen (branched chains of sugar molecules). Muscle insulin fuels the muscles through workout; liver maintains blood glucose, the principal fuel to your brain and nervous system. When blood sugar levels fall because of extended physical action, carbohydrates in the food that we eat could be utilised to generate blood sugar. If the body doesn't get enough carbohydrate throughout the diet, then it is going to make sugar from muscle , a bad choice because the muscular protein is necessary for the task accessible.

Carbohydrate prerequisites

High amounts of constant physical action, for example grinding fireline to get hours, raise the daily caloric needs. Each gram of carbohydrate provides 4 calories .

The following example demonstrates how to calculate the dietary requirement to get a 154-pound firefighter:

Weight (in lbs) 154/ (2.2 pounds/kilogram) = 70 (pounds in kilograms)

Hard function --7 to 10 g of carbohydrate/kilogram/ day x 70 kilograms (body fat) = 490 to 700 g of carbohydrate/day

Throughout work, firefighters require 40 g of carbohydrate every hour out of sport and snacks drinks. A power bar could include 25 grams of carb, and one cup of a sports beverage may include 15 grams, for a total of 40 g of carbohydrate. Field research on firefighters reveal that ingestion carbohydrate enhances function output signal, immune function, blood sugar ability to think clearly mood.

Fat

Fat should offer no greater than 20 to 35 per cent of

daily calories. No more than one third of those fat should come from polyunsaturated and saturated fats (like butter, lard, milk fat, and a few processed fats--browse on the labels). The equilibrium of fat should include polyunsaturated and monounsaturated fats (like olive, canola, and olive oils or out of nuts like almonds, hazelnuts, and olives). When a firefighter requires 4,000 calories every day for significant work, one-quarter may come from fat (1,000 calories). Since each gram of fat contains 9 calories, then that is 111 g (4 oz) of fat daily.

Protein

Trainers and wildland firefighters need 1.2 to 1.8 g of protein per kilogram of body fat every day, together with 1.2 g needed for moderate workout and 1.8 g necessary for protracted challenging work under undesirable conditions. For this particular example, we'll utilize a 154-lb (70-kilogram) firefighter who needs 1.5 g of protein every day for every kilogram of body fat.

1.5 g of protein/kilogram/day x 70 kilograms (body

fat) = 105 g (3.7 oz) of all protein/day.

Electrolytes

Electrolytes are minerals (potassium and sodium) which are significant for nerve/muscle purpose, also for the human body's fluid and also acid/base balances.

To replace electrolytes lost in sweat:

- Utilize the salt shaker at foods

- Eat salty foods (pickles, olives, jerky) during tough function

- Drink carbohydrate/electrolyte beverages (sport drinks) during tough function

- Drink milk at lunch or after work

Sport drinks

Carbohydrate/electrolyte beverages (sport drinks) maintain blood sugar, function output, immune function, disposition, and also the capability to make choices. The electrolytes assist to keep blood circulation and decrease loss of fluid from the urine.

Lightly flavored game beverages promote drinking. To find out more on sport beverages, visit wildland firefighter health and safety report: no. 8 about the mtdc internet website.

Immune function

Psychological stress, fatigue, smoke vulnerability, sleep deprivation, and chamomile may hamper immune function. A balanced diet with sufficient calories, poultry, meat, fruits, and veggies enhances resistance. Studies have shown that eating snacks and drinking game beverages to present additional carbohydrates during function help to keep up the immune purpose of wildland firefighters.

Weight direction

When firing season is finished, consume less as your energy demands will likely be reduced. To shed weight during the off period:

- Boost physical action

- Reduce caloric consumption by

- Decreasing consumption of fats and

sweets

- Decreasing parts of foods

Weigh yourself every two weeks to keep an eye on your progress.

Begin the flame season physically match a solid nutritional foundation.

CHAPTER ONE

BEST DIET FOR FIRE FIGHTERS

As a crisis there's a good deal of doubt once you clock into your change. Actually, just 1 thing is fairly sure - you'll get hungry and need to eat.

Regrettably, as first responders, we're limited to that which we could eat due to active times, lean selection, along with the peer pressure which comes with the land. We need to be mindful of what we're putting in our bodies since our performance could be negatively influenced. It is similar to the analogy goes if you possessed a Lamborghini you would not place the inexpensive fuel right into it, so why do you do the exact same to your own body by filling it with junk foods? In the crisis responders the event the "Lamborghini" can really save people's lives, therefore premium fuel is crucial.

The warrior twenty

The ideal diets and exercise plans are those which

fit best in our lifestyle. Focusing on the ideal foods that are packed with nourishment vitamins, and nutritional supplements can help promote muscle development, psychological longevity, healing, and muscle and cardiovascular endurance.

The subsequent foods are known as the "warrior twenty." all these are the foods which should fill your own kitchen. There is something to be said concerning the true number of unique foods on your fridge. Have a peek in the kitchen of any elite or Olympic athlete and i will ensure the assortment of unique foods that they consume isn't a good deal. So, if you are in the firehouse, the police station, or merely have a cooler on your vehicle, the very same rules must apply. These twenty-five foods can assist you build more muscular, strength, and endurance, and also help reduce a little additional fat.

It may not be the most complicated diet; however, it is simple. Becoming easy makes it simpler to stay with and, even more to the point, sticking with something always makes it a custom. The formulation is even simple, too. The longer you stick with ingesting only these twenty-five meals the greater. Should you include more variety into the twenty-five, then you are going to most probably be moving away from your objective.

Protein

Most individuals do not absorb sufficient protein, that disrupts the muscle building and fixing procedure.

1. Whole eggs: eat entire eggs, not whites. Start looking for the words"free selection, "cage-free," or even"omega-3" in your own egg cartons.

2. Lean meats: chicken, poultry, lean cuts of beef (such as tenderloin), steak, together with wild match (buffalo, venison, elk, ostrich, rabbit).

3. Fatty fish: salmon, sardines, mackerel, and anchovies can help increase mood throughout your lengthy affects and stressful calls.

4. Fermented soy: this creates natural

antibiotic representatives to raise the body's resistance to diseases.

Legumes

These are some excellent sources of fiber, that may help you feel fuller for longer, control blood glucose, and stop cravings when everybody else on your change is becoming second helpings.

5. Beans: little red beans, kidney beans, kidney beans, chick peas, and black beans are all packed with magnesium, iron, magnesium, and potassium.

6. Lentils: low in carbs and ideal for reducing the chances of cardiovascular disease.

Berries

Filled with vitamins, minerals, minerals, and fibers. Seems like mother was onto something when she had to force you to eat all them prior to making the dinner table for a child.

7. Tomatoes: they could help with connective tissue power and help to increase eyesight.

8.	Spinach: filled with vitamin k, that leads to building stronger bones.

9.	Cruciferous vegetables: packing your plate in the firehouse using broccoli, broccoli cabbage, cauliflower, or brussels sprouts may make you feeling fuller more in-between foods.

Berries

Fruits are full of vitamins, minerals, minerals, and fiber like their cousin veggies.

10.	Avocados: studies show that avocadoes can decrease cholesterol and also help you burn off fat.

11.	Citrus fruits: oranges and pineapple are packaged with vitamin c, that can help you stay away from sick days and maintain your immune system in prime shape to help keep you performing at 100 percent.

12.	Berries: raspberries, blueberries, blackberries, berries, and cranberries may continue to keep your memory powerful.

Starches and whole grains

These are the electricity founders. Other diets which have you prevent carbohydrates aren't intended for anybody that has a physical occupation.

13. Sweet potatoes and yams: these behave as your system storage tank for electricity . You have only the correct quantity of energy if you are likely to be battling a fire or following a perp.

14. Quinoa: high in protein, but furthermore, saturated in riboflavin, that has been proven to decrease the frequency of migraines. When there's somebody who copes with sufficient migraines, it is emergency employees.

15. Amaranth: a fantastic way to getting more fiber because it comprises three times greater than wheat.

Healthy fats

Eating the ideal ones will help restrain your hormones, that is essential for obvious reasons.

16. Ingredients: walnuts, almonds, cashews, pecans, and pistachios can help decrease inflammation and also result in a much better mood and psychological procedure. May also be consumed in nut butter type.

17. Seeds: flax, hemp, chia, and berry all include good fats which help you feel fuller for longer.

18. Extra-virgin olive oil: that can be full of antioxidants as well as the healthier monounsaturated fats, that can help control your cholesterol levels.

Drinks

19. Water: water constitutes roughly 70 percent of the body and is essential for each and every metabolic process. I propose carrying out a gallon of water while you're at work, particularly on warm days as soon as your uniform and equipment will enable you to lose additional water than usual.

20. Green tea: a compound in green tea named

egcg can help lower cortisol (your stress hormone) and raise your immune system following long changes.

This warrior twenty is ideal for anybody who has ever fought with diets or finding fantastic equilibrium with their nourishment. By emphasizing foods which you could consume versus avoiding foods which you can't, you are going to increase the prospect of adhering to your diet. This will have a number of advantages - which makes you look great, feel great, and also have a wholesome livelihood.

The impact of sound nutrition on physical functionality, look and wellness are incontrovertible. Simply speaking, if you would like to look, feel and look as a Ferrari, you would better eat a diet full of high-octane foods.

And should you opt to eat as a hog, do not expect to manoeuvre as a gazelle. Nutrition is a crucial bit of the training mystery. Everything you eat is obviously going to boost or hinder your own bodily improvement and functionality.

Give this a notion -- that the next time you wander past a fast-food restaurant, then search at the window and see the outcome of adverse ingestion. Is that where you wish to be? Probably not, particularly if you're studying this novel.

You want to appear good, feel great and perform at the maximum degree. You wish to be more "firefighter match," and also to attain this aim you want to understand to turn into a conscious consumer -- eating correctly, frequently and mild.

You want to eat a performance-oriented diet abundant in"foods which fuel up you and wash out you instead of the ones that slow you down and clog up you. And since you do, you will undoubtedly see the way the body, if properly refrigerated, can do wonders.

This chapter offers you the info that you want to come up with a significant comprehension of healthy and performance-oriented nourishment. Our strategy to performance nourishment is straightforward, demonstrated, sensible and effective.

You will find it simple to comprehend and easy to apply. In learning the fundamental facts and principles that we set forth in these pages, you are going to have the ability to produce high-fat diet a diet that is suitable for your specific preferences and promotes optimum training advancement and functionality.

Straightforward truth #1: your mom was correct it is always pleasant to commence a new segment on a favorable note. Nevertheless, the fantastic news is that the varied, well-balanced and innovative carbohydrate-based diet your mother supplied and insisted that you simply consume has been right on the mark.

She understood of your enormous potential early and consequently fueled one to attain good success from the beginning. Her focus on foods that are whole; fruits, cereals and veggies was utter genius.

She had been your very first good trainer, but it's time to take over the helm and spike ahead. In accord with your mum's instinctive prescription, we advise that you have a diet comprising about 55 to

60 percent carb (mainly complex starches, not simple sugars), approximately 15 per cent protein, and less than 30 per cent fat.

Moreover, you need to certainly reduce your saturated fat intake (less than 10%) and avoid polyunsaturated fatty acids no matter what. Fluid intake must incorporate the bountiful usage of caffeine- and - alcohol-free drinks.

If your diet is nicely balanced (as explained) and really diverse with regard to selected food products, then supplementation using any kind of compound (vitamin, mineral, pre-digested amino acids (magic herbs) is unwarranted.

Having stated that, should you want to fortify your nutrient intake using a fundamental multi-vitamin/multi-mineral for the interest of private assurance or insurance, then go ahead, "no harm, no foul."

Should you keep this equilibrium (55 to 60 percent carbohydrate/roughly 15 per cent protein less compared to 30% fat) and nourish your meals item choice, you're get sufficient amounts of all of the nutrients (like protein) required to prepare and produce optimally. We caution you to not fall prey into the enchanting and slick marketing and advertising efforts of this billion-dollar nutritional supplement market.

Have the suspicious contents out of a huge jar of "nitro-muscle super blaster" (or anything) most surely won't result from the miraculous evolution of monster sized muscles such as people of air-brushed nitro-man, nor can it land you a date with his counterpart nitro woman.

Eating intelligent and training are the methods to get you into where you would like to go -- maybe not some magical potion, powder or tablet computer.

Straightforward truth #2: carbohydrate is the gas to the flame floor carbohydrate is the principal source of gas for firefighting and also the operation of additional high-intensity bodily pursuits. It is also the favourite source of fuel for muscles doing medium to high intensity aerobic function, red blood cells providing oxygen to working muscles, and brain tissues that allow you to think.

Contrary to protein and fat, which is the fuel which eases high-level physical and mental performance in crucial and demanding scenarios. Therefore, to do on the degree of an high-intensity firefighter or high heeled athlete, then you want to eat a carbohydrate-based balanced diet.

Mcardle, pritiken, bailey along with a group of other equally educated nutritionists all urge that vitamin compose the vast majority of your daily caloric consumption. We concur, and for a good reason: it works!

But, recognizing that proportions are often tough to compute though the length of daily, we recommend that you employ the next simple remedy: substitute premium excellent complex carbohydrate foods (vegetables, fruits, cereals, juices and also whole products) for a number of those lower-quality fatty foods you may otherwise tend to consume.

In this doing not only are you going to be loading

your body up with the high energy fuel it needs and needs, but you are also going to be providing it with all the vital vitamins, vitamins, minerals and water it ought to encourage decent health and strength operation.

The more you proceed in the path of whole-food intake, the more quickly you are going to realize the unbelievable fact which you may really eat more and weigh less.

Straightforward truth #3: eat meals which fuel up you and wash you out this simple fact also highlights carbohydrate intake because the usage of complex-carbohydrate foods encourage high end physical functionality, and aids in preventing heart disease and even cancer.

A diet program loaded in (complex) carbohydrates like fruits, vegetables, cereals, grains, juices, pasta and rice supplies you with all the fuel you want to do at your greatest level. Fat, on the other hand, will simply contribute considerably as a supply of gas during the operation of reduced - into moderate-intensity aerobic workout, also nourishment needs to be scavenged in body and then converted into carbohydrate in the liver until it is used as a viable energy supply.

Consequently, foods which are high in protein and fat instead of carbohydrate are very likely to satisfy you up with unusable fuels and also concurrently starve you of this"rocket" fuel that you want to do -- a healthy diet high in fat and protein can let you fatigue faster as unfilled muscle and liver stores of carb fast deplete.

This will possess a negative impact on both the coaching and athletic or firefighting functionality. Warning: high-protein diets are especially harmful to high performance firefighter/athletes.

They neglect to present sufficient carbohydrate fuel and also market the reduction of crucial body fat, electrolyte minerals as well as the fat-soluble vitamins utilized for generating energy. Dehydration can quicken the speed of exhaustion and reduce the body's capability for cooling through high-intensity work or exercise, particularly in hot and humid athletic, instruction and firefighting surroundings.

Thus, swallowing a non-invasive, low-carbohydrate diet which ends in carbohydrate depletion and dehydration can be faulty, unhealthy and possibly deadly for health firefighter/athletes.

CHAPTER TWO

FIRE FIGHTER NUTRITION KEYS TO EFFECTIVE WEIGHT LOSS

The information in NFPA along with other healthcare bureaus is unargued: cardiac cancer and disease are the conflicts which firefighters are confronting --and we're losing. The overall populace is currently fighting a similar battle with coronary artery disease, also in accordance with the centres for disease control and prevention (CDC), 80% of those deaths in this country are preventable. How? What exactly are we doing wrong? Are we losing this battle? Are firefighters losing exactly the exact same fight? The replies have some shared topics but have to be dealt with differently.

Some may have you think that simply doing more movement, more forecasts, more instruction, more exercises your response, and while that's indeed part of the solution, it isn't the complete answer.

Everything you place in your own body as fuel gets a far more profound effect in it than what it is that you're doing with your own body. You can't outwork improper ingestion. Food is gas and we have to know this to fully grasp how to eat exactly what you would like and desire. That doesn't necessarily mean that you can't eat what you like or want to reside on a fast-paced diet plan which you can't sustain to find the scale fall. In reality, both of these choices do not ordinarily result in long-term achievement.

Keeping a wholesome weight along with an active lifestyle is the best way to reduce the possibility of cardiac disease and cancer threat. Lots of firefighters on the occupation have begun have looked at ways to remain healthy by keeping a healthful weight, and also for many that means losing weight reduction having worked with several individuals, including strategic athletes that are well over 400 LBS, I will attest to some basic measures which have to be required to guarantee success.

Ascertain your motivation

To begin with, know why you wish to drop weight. What rationale do you need for trying to make this shift? Since your physician told you also? Since someone made a remark that made you consider doing it? Many people who create this form of shift to please somebody else because they wish to change the way others think or consider them are finally not profitable. That may simply not be sufficient inspiration to create it through the battle of organizing meals, time commitment or even the blank shopping. There has to be an inner incentive private reason this aim is valuable to your general lifetime, not only how that you look or the way others view you, as people are negative effects to the total achievement.

People have different perspectives on how firefighters seem; we make jokes about it. But there's not any denying that if our clients call to our aid, they anticipate high-performing athletes that will physically and emotionally solve issues and threat themselves in hazardous circumstances. Do what you eat affect this skill? It totally can.

Little modifications and easy actions

After knowing the why of fat reduction, then consider how to create it occur. Approaching that is best accomplished by considering what it is you are presently doing. Little sustainable changes can allow you to feel accomplished and also make it something that you simply do versus anything you've changed or do not do. Yes there are those rare men and women that are exceptionally motivated to only make several remarkable life changes adhere, but individuals generally change a lot too quickly and don't feel as they can keep it.

Small adjustments can help with non-scale successes like feeling great about something which is healthy besides simply having the scale fall. By way of instance, challenge yourself to consume more water. A fantastic start is to target for half of an ounce into a complete ounce for every pound of body fat of water daily for another fourteen days. This may have plenty of positive consequences, the significant one being our mind receives signals from our own body on a continuous basis and also the one to get thirst and appetite is all but identical. This usually means that a number of the instances you believe that you're hungry, so you might just be hungry. This could assist with cravings and part sizes. Staying hydrated helps promote circulatory health and enables your joints and muscles work better.

As significant as it is to remain hydrated, that can't be the only real change you make if losing weight is the objective. In regards to ingestion, you will find so many ways which operate for specific body types and lifestyles, however, there are some great tips and information that can help with most of these:

eliminate processed sugar in your own intake. This will aid your blood glucose levels equilibrium, help in weight reduction, reduce fat , reduce empty calorie consumption.

eat fresh foods foods which aren't heavily processed, like fruits, veggies, grains, oats, animal meats, etc.,.

quit eating 2-3 hours. Occasionally this can be

challenging for people who don't sleep much because of large call volume. For those people, it may be about which sort of food you're eating versus when you're eating it. When it's the center of the evening and you are coming back in a run, prevent considerable quantities of carbs and attempt to maintain your consumption concentrated on fresh protein resources or a fast little snack which isn't heavy in carbohydrates.

substitute whole wheat and whole grain selections for the white. By way of instance, using breads, rice and pasta, the brown material is best for fat loss compared to the white things.

earn more than you want and save for later.

Meal prep

For this last suggestion, many who are trying weight reduction are knowledgeable about this term"meal preparation," that is essentially making meals in bulk to be consumed afterwards. Individuals who are able to master this ability normally see superior results in weight reduction.

When you're making foods that are targeted toward weight reduction, be enough that you're able to consume it for a different one, a couple of meals at the moment. After all, time is among the largest hurdles in weight reduction --insufficient time to visit the shop, insufficient time to produce healthful meals, insufficient time to stay with this. So, not to squander time, the majority of the foods you consume should be considered, carefully planned and prepared beforehand.

This tends to be the toughest thing for individuals to focus on however also by way the best in reducing your weight. That is a place where you only have to commit the time to generate the meals beforehand to ensure yourself a meal that is clean. Then, stay with it. This isn't something which see's remarkable shift in a couple weeks or even 21 days. This may take some time and effort, however just like most things in your life, you'll get from this what you put in it.

Let us be blunt: quick fixes don't work. No diet pill in the marketplace will make you eliminate fat without changing your nourishment too. Fad diets and diet programs may take off some weight, however if they're not healthful sustainable strategies for long-term achievement, they'll fail also. Quit seeking the easy way out, there's not anything that will provide you the success you're interested in finding out of the tough job of eating correctly (the majority of the time) and remaining busy (all time). Here is what will add quality years to everything you could do to the occupation and many years on to a life once you retire, interval. Thus, you have to be aware it is well worth it, and you're worth the effort it takes.

Professional advice

When it comes to the things to eat and when to eat it, then that differs from individual to individual when weight reduction is your objective. I suggest getting some expert assistance, like a nutritionist, gym, trainer or someone who can assist you in making the proper decisions for you, browse the metrics and know that your results. Why? Because not all of weight is made equal. When weight reduction is your goal, it's extremely imperative that you're monitoring fat reduction, not only weight loss. This is the area where nutrition can play a much larger role in relation to exercise.

Body fat, especially visceral and subcutaneous fat, is a lot detrimental to our wellbeing. If you're losing considerable quantities of fat , your system is experiencing a process of losing weight aside from fat, since it seems it's hungry so the scale might fall, however you'll notice that you don't feel well, along with the pounds will struggle to return on.

An instrument such as a human body or a digital body fat step is an excellent way to monitor the kind of weight you're losing. Should you choose your own leg and multiply it from your own body fat percent as a match, then you'll become about the number of pounds of fat will be in your own body now. Just take that number and then subtract it out of your overall body fat and you'll have an approximate number of fat muscle. These figures aren't accurate, but that is a powerful approach to quantify results past the scale.

The quantity of body weight that you need to carry differs among sex and age. For example, the american college of sports medicine imply that men between age 30 to 39 keep a body fat percent under 20.4 percent and girls in precisely the exact same age range under 24.8 percent.

Support methods

Past the expert advice, other service methods, for example family and colleagues, are critical for success. Let your colleagues know that you're focusing on bettering yourself, but not just for the task but also for the men and women who sit alongside you about the vehicle. Let them understand how they could assist, and discuss your strategy in order that they may help keep you accountable. It is likely that they will be inclined to encourage you however they could. As firefighters, we are apt to keep away from getting the weight reduction dialog due to the anxiety of individuals feeling attacked . However, this isn't private; this can be specialist. The requirements of the project are the requirements of this project, the information is the information. We will need to care about our occupation and the men and women who take action to have this challenging conversation. It is not any different than every other portion of the task. In the event that you needed a firefighter who may not correctly utilize a saw or progress a hoseline, then we'd work together till they had the ability to perform it.

We love the term "brotherhood," but should we actually mean it, then these would be the discussions that have to occur, since it is killing firefighters. We are not speaking about discussions that strike people but instead conversations that allow the individual understand that you attention, and you're inclined to assist.

What exactly does that look like? As a change, possess a performance mindset, either with trainings which you're doing along with the fuel you're putting into your system. Shop and consume the way you need your body to do on a significant incident. When creating dishes together, create them from actual ingredients and create health-conscious choices. Have trained speakers and we come in and current trainings and plans which you could apply at your section. Enable your wellbeing and safety committee to make decisions according to a general aim for the whole department. Deliver health-passionate firefighters to conventions, train-the-trainers and conventions to bring thoughts back which could do the job for your section, then have an open mind on it rather than shutting it down since it differs from everything you've done previously.

Fight the battle

We have to stop treating our devices better compared to our firefighters. We strive so difficult to execute continuous maintenance checks and clean-up, and place appropriate fuel and money into our devices, but the men and women who ride from the device are a lot more useful and significant to our general aim. This will be a difficult struggle, but it's well worth it, our folks are worthwhile, and incorporating quality years on somebody's life with people they love is well worth everything it takes.

Fight the battle and know you've got people.

CHAPTER THREE

5 NUTRITION HACKS FOR FIREFIGHTERS

There is a popular slogan in the fitness sector that "you cannot out-exercise a lousy diet" eating pizza, with a beer and ending with a few ice cream sounds excellent, but it won't help you work or seem better about the fire and save scene irrespective of how much you work out. Sure that diet might have functioned for you once you're 17, but since you get older, your metabolism slows, and you have probably realized a greater performance and body begins from the kitchen.

Eating from the firehouse--or should i say, eating healthful at the firehouse--could be a really tough endeavour. There's generally plenty of baked products out of grateful citizens and very fantastic hamburgers. Cooking at the firehouse is much harder. Cook something healthful and hear it in the team. Cook something yummy and it is probably full of fat and calories. This normally contributes to large portions and surplus food for after meals.

But all isn't lost. There are just five easy nourishment tips that will assist you stay healthy and maintain your weight in check.

1. Out of sight out of thoughts

If you walk to many firehouse kitchens, then you're usually greeted with. Sweet scents and the sight of fresh baked goods and candy. Typically, you likely are not overly hungry, but since those goodies are facing you, you're more inclined to indulge. I understand the firehouse civilization would rip you apart if you're that person to really throw these bites. But that does not mean that you can not set them in a cabinet or in the refrigerator. Let us face it, even if it's out of sight, then it's out of the mind. I'd also go a step farther and put some new veggies or fruit to the desk. You might find some backlash initially, but diminishing the temptation is well worth it.

2. Drink it up (water, which is)

Among the most important things you can do for improved nutrition and a successful diet is drink sufficient water. Water is the crucial element to many metabolic functions within the human body, such as digestion and removal. Staying hydrated will assist with functionality, decrease your odds of sudden cardiac arrest and strokes, and also can help you suppress your hunger. Just how much water should you consume a day? An overall recommendation is to consume eight 8-oz. Cups of water daily for a total of 64 ounce. This ought to be the minimal for firefighters. This amount goes up in the event that you work out, work at a hot weather, or even possess a passion call in which you eliminate a great deal of fluid. And do not hesitate to feel thirsty to begin drinking water.

3. Eat your veggies and fruits

Veggies and fruits must be included in each meal and in as many snacks as possible. They supply the body with muscle building and energy-promoting nutrients a firefighter should make it through daily. By mixing your system with the largest possible quantity of nourishment to the number of calories, they're a dietary deal. If the fruit or veggie in question will not rust after a couple of days of hanging out around the counter, then then it is a processed meals. Be certain you choose leafy, green, lower-starch vegetables over starchier kinds. Some instances include broccoli, lettuce, cauliflower, cabbage and lettuce. Starchier kinds comprise potatoes, yams and sweet potatoes.

4. Reduce tooth

It appears to be a frequent staple in any firehouse, much more so on the vacations --donuts around the desk, snacks on the counter tops and ice cream in the refrigerator. However, since it is there does not mean that you ought to always indulge. It has been well documented that glucose may have a detrimental impact on your health. Studies have linked this candy chemical to obesity, cardiovascular disease, liver disease, greater levels of cancer, and tooth decay alongside different issues. Sugar also has an addictive quality which makes it a difficult"custom" to split. Start reading labels. Sugar is hidden and it frequently replaces fat from low-fat/fat-free meals, and you're going to discover it in things which may truly be produced from only a couple of ingredients such as nut butters, breads and salad dressings. Check nutrition labels that will assist you decide on the meals without added sugar or opt for the low-sugar edition. Rather than sugary, carbonated beverages and juice beverages (pop up), choose water or unsweetened tea. Should you choose sugar in hot beverages or add it into cereal, then slowly lower the amount before you may cut it out. Additionally, reduce desserts in amount or frequency. It is ok to indulge sometimes, but attempt to obey portion sizes when you're doing. It could be hard initially to lower your sugar consumption, but once you do, i promise you will start to see a difference in how that you feel.

5. Head your parts

Many firehouses not just serve plenty of food, however they generally function them on big plates. Let us be fair, it will feel too great to fill your plate when you are hungry at the conclusion of the day. But if you are fighting to finish it all or you are feeling a massive energy slump following your meal, then it is likely to be an indication that you are getting more food than your body requires. A very simple change of dinnerware size might be a remarkably handy remedy to the huge firehouse functioning size. Research indicates that people eat around 22 percent fewer calories if they are in a position to lower the total amount of empty space in their plate.one fundamentally, when you find a massive plate with vacant emptiness round the meals, the mind unconsciously presumes the plate comprises significantly less food than the usual smaller-sized dish without a white area. Hence the important thing is to function your firehouse meals on smaller plates. Rather than employing a large 14-inch plate to your foods, elect to get an 8-inch plate. If you are using distinct plates for various foods, then you can change things around to your benefit. Use bowls for salads and veggies and smaller dishes to the grains and meat. And do not return for seconds. It requires your mind everywhere from 20 to 30 minutes to indicate your belly is complete, therefore slow down your eating. You're most likely complete and do not understand it yet!

It requires dedication

Whether you're cooking or just eating at the firehouse (or some other home), those food hacks will help but you must use them. Wholesome nutrition takes some preparation and dedication. The effort is well worth it. Eat better, do better and better.

Nutrition is a crucial part of the health and security of wildland fire suppression staff. This can be the fuel for your body to execute the function and preserve cognitive skills. Wildland firefighters around the fire line require 4,000-6,000 calories per day to never enter an energy shortage.

Think about the following key factors when selecting your meal:

- There are just three big energy resources in foods: protein, carbs, and carbohydrates.

- Carbohydrates (also referred to as sugar) provide a direct supply of energy to the human body. They supply the fuel to the muscles and organs, like your mind.

- Proteins are the fundamental building blocks of the body. They comprise of amino acids which help build muscles, skin, blood, hair, nails and internal organs.

- Fat is a vital nutrient that offers energy, energy storage, insulation, and shape to your system.

- Mtdc urges ingestion 150-200 kcals every two hours throughout the work shift to keep blood sugar levels and energy levels.

Carbohydrates:

- Studies athletes have revealed that carbs are the most crucial energy supply for functionality and wellness.

- Carbohydrates are the body's first selection for fuel. If given a choice of many kinds of foods concurrently, your own body will utilize the energy from carbs .

- In case you don't eat enough carbs, the following may happen:

- Fatigue.

- Muscle cramps.

- Poor psychological function.

- The flame camp lunches (known as change food) are intended to permit firefighters small quantities of food (mostly carbohydrates) which is readily eaten during the work shift.

CHAPTER FOUR

WHAT'S THE ENGINE TWO DIET?

The engine two meals concentrates on mostly unprocessed plant-based foods . Along with removing animal products, the engine two meals is low fat and absolutely free from vegetable oils. Followers of this diet eat whole foods such as legumes, fruits, grains, vegetables, nuts, and legumes. Though the engine two meals can assist in weight reduction, it is not especially a weight reduction program. Instead, the diet promotes overall well-being.

Wallpaper

The engine two diet was made by rip esselstyn, a former practitioner athlete, also firefighter. His dad, dr. Caldwell esselstyn, is a doctor and physician that promotes a diet to stop and reverse cardiovascular disease. After he became a firefighter, then rip esselstyn chose his enthusiasm to get a plant-based diet into the firehouse. He aided his colleagues enhance their health using a diet plan surrounded by complete, unprocessed foods with very little fat.

Rip esselstyn turned into a bestselling writer if he shared his trip knowledge from the publication"the engine two meals " after helping his fellow firefighters reach a course to enhance well-being, he wished to assist americans confronting similar health issues.

The engine two meals does not highlight weight reduction, but instead focuses on decreasing cholesterol levels, preventing heart disease and getting a"plant-strong" person.

The way it works

The engine two meals have very definite guidelines. You're expected to remove all animal products and vegetable oils. The diet is made of low-carb meals which are created chiefly with foods that are unprocessed.

Things to eat

Compliant foods

legumes

whole grains

fruits

vegetables

seeds and grains

 non-dairy milk

tofu and tempeh

engine two meals line-up

Non-compliant foods

animal goods

citrus oils

processed foods

processed vegan meals

added sugar and salt

high-calorie fluids

Legumes

Savory foods with this diet frequently incorporate

legumes such as lentils and legumes. You are invited to create certain the beans are oil-free and low-sodium. Stock on black beans, pinto beans, chickpeas, red lentils, brown peas, split peas and so forth.

Whole grains

Engine two isn't a low-carb diet, so you can enjoy brown rice with your lunch or dinner. Other grains include oats, quinoa, and amaranth. It is possible to also have pasta, cereal, and bread on the engine two meals provided that they are 100% whole grain.

Fruits

Fruit is compliant about the engine two meals, however, there are a number of ground rules. Fruit needs to be frozen or fresh. This usually means no dehydrated cherry, raisinsand banana chips, etc.. The main reason being is that dehydrated fruit frequently has added fat, sugar, and carbs. You also have to consume fruit in its complete form, and thus don't mix it. It is advised that you use fruit into high your foods, like adding berries and blueberries for your morning oatmeal.

Berries

Considering that the engine two meals urges low-fat foods, vegetables are a staple. Rip esselstyn recommends supplementing meals up with leafy greens because they are low in carbs and high in nutrition. It's possible to delight in both cooked and raw veggies onto the engine two meals. Starchy vegetables such as potatoes are also contained in the meal program.

Nuts and seeds

Instead of snacking on nuts and seeds, then the engine two meals utilizes them as condiments. As an instance, you may add chia seeds into your oatmeal and chopped almonds into your salad. Proceed to get raw, unsalted nuts and seeds, even however, to prevent extra oil and salt.

Non-dairy coffee

Plant milk is permitted on the engine two meals. Take your choice from milk, soy milk, almond milk, rice milk, oat milk and much more. Just be certain it's unsweetened as numerous non-dairy milks are sweetened with glucose.

Tofu and tempeh

A fantastic way to put in protein to the engine two meals would be using tofu and tempeh. Steer clear of those which are either pre-seasoned or marinated since they are likely high in salt, sugar, and fatloss.

Engine two food line

The engine two meals includes its own food lineup available only at whole foods market. The line contains cereal, wheat burgers, plant milks, vegetable stock, granola, soup, hummus, pasta, burritos and much more. What's vegan, low-sodium, oil-free, low-sugar and low-carb.

Animal products

In its heart, the engine two meals is a expansion of this vegan diet. You may replace animal products and services. This usually means removing food groups: animal protein and milk.

Vegetable oils

Removing oils cuts the number of calories you are consuming. The engine two meals is oil-free and does not make exceptions to olive oil, coconut oil or other oils that are generally associated with being healthful fats.

Refined foods

You will notice that the engine two meals urges whole foods like wheat bread rather than white bread. Processed foods such as bread, cereal, and bread are also reduced in fiber high in carbs. Whole-grain options are suggested to help keep you feeling fuller for more than one.

Processed vegan food

Vegan food is not inherently healthy. There are infinite options available on the marketplace for sausage nuggets, macn' cheese, ice cream, cakes, etc.. When these foods are vegan, they are not engine two compliant since they are usually high in carbs, sugar, fat, sodium, and petroleum.

Additional salt and sugar

A frequent mistake people get on the engine two

meals is including sugar and salt to foods. When purchasing canned and boxed products including canned beans and instant yoghurt, be sure they are low-sodium and sugar-free.

High-calorie liquids

The engine two meals features a firm position against consuming your calories. This means that you should just drink plain water, black coffee, and green tea. Jump on smoothies, vegetable and fruit juices, soda pop and other drinks that are high in sugar and calories. By ingesting calorie-free drinks, you may obviously have fewer calories.

Recommended timing

The engine two meals requires for three chief meals: breakfast, dinner, lunch, and lunch). There aren't any dedicated snacks with this diet program. You'll have snacks in the event that you'd like so long as they stick to the very same principles that foods follow.

Resources and tips

The official engine two diet site offers a free 7-day

challenge plus a catalogue of recipes.

If you do not have time to prepare new foods, rip esselstyn urges the engine two meals exclusively offered in whole sale foods market.

The engine two meals is not free of allergens. It is obviously free of milk, eggs, and shellfish, however, it includes additional pollutants, such as soy, soy free and tree nuts. If you are allergic to those foods, then it's possible to just omit them in the engine two meals.

Considering that the diet plan is free of animal products, you might need to take vitamin d. And vitamin b12 nutritional supplements. As an alternative, you can eat compliant foods which are fortified such as almond milk along with supplements.

Pros and cons

emphasizes whole foods

 no calorie counting

high in fiber

promotes heart health

could be used for weight loss loss

Disadvantages

restrictive

folks may experience migraines

engine two meals line is pricey

emphasizes whole foods

Nearly all engine two foods are made out of whole, unprocessed foods. Consuming whole foods is also an significant part the diet since it enables followers to eat lots of micronutrients.

No calorie counting

Many diets need followers to rigorously monitor their calories macronutrient ingestion. There is zero relying on this diet program.

High fiber

Possessing a high-fiber diet includes lots of wellbeing advantages . Fiber is very important to digestion and also keeps you fuller for longer. The engine two meals is high in fiber since it's all plant-based.

Promotes heart health

The engine two diet initially began as a strategy for neighborhood firefighters to lower your cholesterol. It was produced with center health in your mind as heart disorder is the major killer.

May be used to weight loss

While weight loss is not the principal aim of this engine two meals, followers may shed weight. The diet plan is low carb and obviously lower in carbs, therefore weight reduction with this diet plan is potential.

Disadvantages

Restrictive

The engine two meals is significantly more restrictive than a normal plant-based diet . A vegetarian diet is currently free from animal products, however engine two carries it a step farther. Followers must remove sugar and oil. They need to also reduce fat and salt.

Individuals may expertise cravings

When diets are somewhat restrictive, folks can be more prone to get cravings. The engine two meals does not have snacks assembled into the program, so this can increase cravings, also.4

Engine two food line is expensive

While not mandatory, people after this diet can buy and eat engine two branded food items out of whole foods market. Nonetheless, these goods are more costly compared to other foods allowed in your diet program. By way of instance, a 2-pack of engine two teaspoons burgers is 4.99.

How it compares

The engine two meals is like most diet, but engine two is more rigorous in regards to vegetable oils and other nutritional supplements. There are foods that remove animal products, for instance, macrobiotic diet, raw food diet, diet and fruitarian diet. But, those diets vary in engine two because they highlight specific food groups.

Usda tips

The 2015-2020 usda dietary guidelines admit that vegetarians and vegans can fulfill nutrient needs without animal products. On the other hand, the guidelines imply that meatless diets are generally reduced in vitamin d. Considering that the engine two meals is a healthy diet, followers must monitor their consumption of vitamin b-12vitamin d, along with other nutrients.3

Limited calories

With restricted vegetable oils and resources of protein and fat, the engine two diet is low in carbs. The guidelines do not need followers to rely on calories, therefore there are not some dietary recommendations.

Individuals who wish to eliminate weight could do this with this diet because it consists of low-carb foods such as leafy greens, legumes, beans, and veggies. However, those who seem to the diet plan to enhance their heart health should make certain they are ingesting a large enough quantity of meals to meet their caloric requirements.

Limited nutrients

Like other kinds of vegetarian diets, the engine two meals which makes it more challenging to have specific nutrients.

For sufficient protein to the engine two meals, make certain to eat a protein origin in foods. Seeds and grains may add more protein into your morning oats, and beans can raise the quantity of protein on your dinner and lunch foods.

Fruits and vegetables are high in several micronutrients, but vitamins b-12 and d may be challenging. Followers are counseled to eat fortified foods such as engine two cereal along with non-dairy milk. Nutritional supplements are also an alternative.

The engine two meals is not the only diet which eliminates animal products. There are additional vegan diets on the market. Some diets are more restrictive while some are more lenient. See the way the engine two meals contrasts.

Engine two diet

1. What's: the engine two meals is a strict vegan diet. It is made of mostly whole, unprocessed plant foods. Followers remove animal products, vegetable oils and also extra sugar. They need to also decrease their fat and salt consumption. Though the engine two meals helps people eliminate weight, its principal objective is to help individuals lower their cholesterol and protect against cardiovascular disease.

2. Security: this nutritional supplement presents no dangers as long as folks are fulfilling their needs for nourishment and a few micronutrients.

3. Sustainability: in concept, this diet could be sustained long term. But it is quite rigorous and followers create experience cravings which make them drift from the diet program. Additionally, it is tough to eat at restaurants with this diet

program.

Macrobiotic diet

1. What's: much like the engine two meals, the most macrobiotic diet is full of fiber and low in fat loss. Additionally, it is mostly plant-based, but a few followers eat fish sometimes. Contrary to the engine two meals, the macrobiotic could be adjusted to satisfy the requirements of people based on age, age, sex and activity level and much more.

2. Security: this diet is also full of macronutrients and micronutrients. But, experts warn that nutritional deficiencies might happen with this diet as it limits some food collections. Much like the engine two meals, lovers of the macrobiotic diet have been invited to guarantee they're consuming dietary resources of particular nutrients.

3. Sustainability: the macrobiotic is

designed to be a lifelong diet plan. On the other hand, the prohibitive nature of this diet might be hard for individuals in their daily lives.

Raw food diet

1. What's: the raw food concentrates mostly on foods in their raw form. Even though some folks include raw animal products, it is mainly a vegetarian diet.

2. Security: though this particular diet is filled with micronutrients, it is nutritionally incomplete and introduces several dangers. Folks are in danger of vitamin b-12 lack. Girls are more inclined to come up with amenorrhea (the absence of menstruation).

3. Sustainability: removing cooked meals is unsustainable. Followers of the diet are known to eat cooked meals on event or revert into a diet that frequently incorporates cooked meals.

Fruitarian diet

1. What's: the fruitarian diet is just what it resembles. Followers of the diet have fruit for as many as 90 percent of the foods. They might also eat seeds, nuts, and a few veggies.

2. Security: possessing fruit has many added benefits, but also the fruitarian diet lacks diversity. Experts think that followers of the diet confine themselves from additional protein and fat resources.

3. Sustainability: this nutritional supplement is unsustainable since fruit is low in protein and calories. Fruit can also be expensive to stay off.

CHAPTER FIVE

WHAT TO EXPECT ON A VEGAN DIET?

Vegan diets and other healthful eating styles are becoming popular as the health and ecological advantages they provide are becoming more evident. A growing amount of studies correlate long-term ingestion with favourable health effects, such as a decreased risk of cardiovascular disease, type two diabetes, stroke, diabetes and other health ailments. If you are thinking about adopting a vegetarian way of life, think about the modifications you would have to create to your present diet plan, shopping, and dinner customs before determining if it's ideal for you.

Things to eat

A vegan diet excludes all animal products. With this particular eating program, not only would you prevent any foods that comes straight from an animal source, but also you avoid any foods which has any creature by-product within it.

Compliant foods

vegetables

fruit

grains

legumes

seeds and grains

soy-based goods

plant-based oils

Non-compliant foods

beef and poultry

fish and fish

eggs

dairy goods

honey

animal by-products

Compliant foods

Berries

In a vegetarian diet, vegetables play an important part. Eating a wide array of vibrant vegetables can allow you to attain your everyday nutrient needs when you consume based on a vegetarian food program.

Collard greens and okra, for

Example, are full of calcium--a nutritional supplement that's essential for vegans since they steer clear of dairy. Spinach, kale, broccoli, brussels sprouts, and broccoli supply nourishment alongside other nutrients.

Vegetables are usually used instead of beef from traditional dishes like lasagna, casseroles, soup. They may also be used to substitute conventional starchy foods which may include non-vegan ingredients. By way of instance, some cooks make noodles from zucchini or like non-dairy mashed cauliflower rather than mashed potatoes made out of milk and butter.

Fruit

Fruit supplies healthful fiber and other nutrients that

are important to some vegan diet. Strawberries, by way of instance, offer calcium, calcium, folate, and potassium. And fiber-rich raspberries are a fantastic source of potassium and vitamin c.

Fruit is also used to replace other foods which are trivial in other diets. By way of instance, bananas may be utilized rather than eggs to earn two-ingredient pancakes. Frozen fruit can be zest, whipped, and rooted to be appreciated within an ice-cream replacement.

On a vegetarian diet, then you spend time searching preparing or for meat, milk, or seafood solutions. This leaves more time for one to experiment with various kinds of vegetables and fruits. Filled with exotic fruits or uncommon vegetables can help to maintain variety in your daily life diet. Eating more whole fruits and veggies may also allow you to reduce your reliance on processed vegan foods, such as veggie chips, imitation meat products, and packaged products.

Grains

Whole grains play an integral part in a healthy diet. Both elegant grains and whole grains have been well balanced on a vegetarian diet, however, picking whole grains can allow you to get to your preferred intake of nutrients that are important -- particularly protein.

Quinoa, by way of example, is a full protein . That usually means it includes all eight essential amino acids. These are amino acids that have to be absorbed in the diet because the body does not make them. Other high-protein grains contain amaranth, oats, wild rice, and buckwheat.

Whole grains also provide fiber and minerals such as vitamin b, e, and folic acid along with important minerals like magnesium, zinc, and iron.

Legumes

Legumes, such as legumes, beans, and lentils, are more healthy, cheap, flexible, and simple to shop. Legumes are low in fat and supply fiber, protein, and other nutrients such as folate, potassium, magnesium, and iron. Legumes also include resistant starch that kind of starch that isn't digested in the gut but instead goes right into the large intestine where it feeds healthful bacteria.

Because beans can easily be added to salads, soups, along with other dishes that they create a wise substitute for meat should you stick to a vegetarian diet.

Nuts and seeds

Seeds and grains can be a fantastic source of protein and healthy fat at a vegan diet. Additionally, foods produced from seeds and nuts may replace foods which aren't compliant within a vegetarian diet. By way of instance, nut butters may substitute milk butter or other stalks, vegan cheese is occasionally produced from nuts (for instance, cashews or almonds) and virtually every supermarket sells milk choices generated from almonds, macadamia nuts, cashews, and other nuts.

Soy-based products

Soy beans and soy products are usually consumed at a vegetarian diet. Edamame--soybeans which aren't yet older --are usually boiled, salted and consumed strategy. Mature soybeans could be consumed and roasted as a snack or used as an ingredient in other foods.

Soy-based foods include broccoli, tempeh, and soy milk. You will also find soy-based yogurt goods, soy ice cream, soy milk powders, and soy protein bars. But not each processed soy product is vegan, therefore it's crucial to look at the ingredients list should you abide by a strict vegetarian diet.

Plant-based oils

Plant-based oils contain olive oil, coconut oil, olive oil, jojoba oil, and lots of more. When these oils contain nine calories per gram such as other fats, they supply monounsaturated and polyunsaturated fat. Beef and dairy products contain less fat that is saturated.

Unsaturated fats are usually liquid at room temperature and are connected to many health benefits such as decreased cholesterol levels, a decrease chance of cardiovascular disease, and decreased risk for stroke.

Non-compliant foods

Beef and poultry

A primary distinction between a vegetarian diet and a standard american diet is that the lack of poultry and meat. While traditional japanese foods are constructed around meat normally using vegetables and starchy foods inserted side dishes, even a vegetarian diet eradicates this crucial component altogether.

Some vegans remove poultry and meat in the diet to encourage animal rights or for ecological factors. Others do this for health reasons. Eliminating poultry and meat in the diet gets rid of a key supply of carbs and saturated fat. Various studies have proven that vegans have a tendency to eat fewer calories and less saturated fat compared to those who eat both animal and plant foods.

Steak and fish

Fish and fish are likewise not have on a vegetarian diet. There may be various reasons for this option, however, a few vegans feel that fish ingestion promotes animal cruelty in precisely the exact same manner that animal ingestion does. Others are worried about the effects of industrial fishing on the surroundings. And a few are concerned about the existence of toxins, like mercury and polychlorinated biphenyls (industrial goods or compounds, also known as bcps). Based the national oceanic and atmospheric administration (noaa), bcps are prohibited since 1979 but might nevertheless be present in deserts, resulting in concerns about their effect on human wellbeing.

Eggs

Eggs can also be off-limits after consuming a vegetarian diet. There are some moral concerns from the community (and elsewhere) regarding the custom of egg farming. Others are worried about the saturated fat content.

Since eggs are a main component in baked goods, pasta, pasta, sauces, as well as other frequent foods it's very important to read labels to ensure the products that you select a vegetarian diet do not include them.

Dairy

Cheese, cheese, cheese and other dairy goods aren't absorbed on a vegan diet. Additionally, foods produced with these components aren't consumed. But if you're a dairy enthusiast, you will discover quite a couple of dairy replacements in the regional sector. Milk, cheese, cheese, and yogurt options can be produced from soy or nuts. Again, it's necessary to read labels. Some products include whey or casein as components and those really are by-products of the milk.

Honey

There's some debate about the usage of bee products, such as honey on a vegetarian diet. Some vegans feel that because bees are creatures and animal products must be prevented, then honey is still really a food that is sour. Yet, others think that because bees aren't harmed from the assortment of honey and because most insects are employed in the farming of crops, it's sensible to absorb honey.

Animal by-products

If you're a whole-food vegetarian, then you certainly do not have to be overly concerned about animal-based ingredients into your meals. But if you consume processed vegan foods, then you are going to need to read ingredient labels carefully to be certain your food does not incorporate some creature by-product.

By way of example, gelatin (generally utilized to make fruit dyes, pudding, candy, etc.. Marshmallows, cakes, ice cream, and yoghurt) is created by boiling skin, ligaments, tendons, or bones of creatures. Other animal-based components to search for contain whey, casein, lactose, egg whites, fish-derived omega-3 fatty acids, rennet, and also a few sorts of vitamin d3.

Recommended timing

There's not any particular meal time consuming practice connected with a vegetarian diet. But if you're thinking about moving into a vegetarian diet by a classic american diet, then the timing of your own transition can affect your success.

Eliminating familiar and foundational foods (such as milk and meat) in the diet may result in feelings of appetite, frustration, as well as disappointment. If you get overwhelmed, then you might stop before learning how to take pleasure in the vegan way of life.

Remember you don't need to adopt a vegetarian eating program all at one time. Some specialists advise that you embrace a flexitarian diet. A flexitarian diet is really a modified vegetarian diet which permits you to consume meat on a few restricted events. As soon as you're familiar with all the flexitarian eating mode, it is possible to completely embrace a vegetarian diet then eventually go vegan.

Another approach that might help ease the transition would be that the "add, subtract later" strategy. In accordance with the process, you begin to add pleasing vegetarian dishes into your own menu prior to subtracting foods which are non-compliant. You remove the foods you're dependent on last--if your own vegan eating strategy has a solid basis.

Resources and tips

A vegetarian diet requires much more work once you first start, only because you need to become thoughtful in your purchasing, cooking, and meal preparation customs. In the supermarket, by way of instance, finding foods which are 100% vegetarian demands the attentive reading of food labels.

Combining carbohydrates

There's a longstanding belief that to be able to become a healthy veganfoods must be carefully blended to provide whole protein. This idea is obsolete since we know a few things about protein we all did not understand previously.

As an example, plant foods contain all the amino acids people desire, both those who we have to eat in the diet (since our bodies do not create them) and also the ones that are non-essential (our own bodies create them). Amino acids are well thought of as building material such as complex amino acids, and people, then, will be the building blocks for virtually everything our bodies will need to build on daily basis: hormones, enzymes, and cells.

Plant foods change at the levels of amino acids. Therefore, by way of example, grains are usually low in the amino acid lysine, however full of cysteine. Beans are high in cysteine, however rich in lysine. Consuming free plant-based foods generates a complete meeting of amino acids at almost deal percentages. And contrary to popular belief, it's not essential that each one of those amino acids--or even building materials--arrive in precisely the exact same time to construct a healthful body.

Even the vegetarian resource group provides a graph of some of those vegetarian or vegan labels you might find on goods in the shop. The chart offers detailed information regarding the criteria used to rate food components and whether food makers are billed for supplying the tag.

For many users, eating whole foods and attentively studying labels will offer the best assurance that their food options align with their vegetarian eating fashion. Rather than relying upon front-of-package product asserts, read the ingredients list to be certain no fish, poultry, or animal by-products are all utilized to create it.

Cooking and planning meals

As soon as you have your carefully chosen vegan foods in your home, you may find out about cook and prepare vegetarian foods by experimenting with new recipes, attempting new sweeteners and spices, and branching out using fresh veggies, seeds, nuts, and walnuts.

Portobello mushroom burgers, by way of example, really are a satisfying replacement for beef hamburgers. Utilizing peanuts or cashews rather than fish or poultry at a stir fry aids make your meal filling and flavorful.

Pros and cons of a vegan diet

A vegetarian diet is a vegetarian eating style, however it is totally devoid of animal products, such as honey, eggs, and dairy goods. Some vegans pick the diet to health reasons, while others favor it for moral reasons, like preventing animal cruelty and swallowing more foods that are sustainable.

While there are documented health benefits of a vegetarian diet, a few find that the lifestyle hard to keep. Consider each one of the advantages and disadvantages of a vegetarian diet until you decide if it's the ideal application for you.

evidence-based health advantages

encourages cautious eating

wider assortment of meals

may cause weight reduction

reduced food prices

healthier for your own surroundings

no creature impact

Disadvantages

restricted food choices

potential nutrient deficiencies

requires diligence

difficulty dining outside

unrealistic expectations

social isolation

The reason (or reasons) which you opt for a vegetarian eating program will decide the advantages which are most important to you personally. But benefits to the lifestyle are significant, whether or not you're picking it for environmental, health, or moral factors.

Health benefits

Since a vegetarian diet is wholesome, it is simpler to load up on healthful whole grains, legumes, vegetables, and veggies that lots of individuals on regular diets deficiency. Studies comparing several kinds of diets have discovered that vegetarian eating rankings best for nutrient excellent. A vegetarian diet is usually high in fiber, calcium, vitamin c, calcium, iron, calcium, and folate and reduced in saturated fats and saturated fats.

The nutrient quality of a vegetarian diet contributes to more substantial wellness advantages. Eating a diet full of foods that are fermented has long been associated with a diminished risk of several chronic ailments. A large cohort study assessed vegetarian and vegetarian diets. Researchers discovered that both groups experienced a lower risk of cardiovascular ailments, cardiometabolic risk factors, several cancers, and overall mortality. People who have been vegan appreciated those benefits together with a decreased risk of hypertension, obesity, type-2 diabetes, and cardiovascular disease.

Additional research have verified those findings also have discovered that plant-based eating might assist in the management and treatment of elevated blood pressure, cardiovascular disease, and eye disease.

Mindful eating

Mindful eating is an exercise which entails paying additional attention to our meals and raising sexual awareness and expertise with a meal. It requires that the eater to be emptied intentionally on ingestion behaviour to relish the practice of ingestion instead of any particular nutritional result (carbs, protein, fat, carbs). Mindful eating habits are correlated with a much healthier relationship with food and also have been utilized in certain weight loss interventions.

Vegan ingestion and mindful ingestion are distinct. However, since vegan eaters want to be mindful and aware in their food options, specific mindful eating habits are made in their meal preparation.

For instance, if you have a conventional american diet, it's easy to catch a meal on the move at a fast-food restaurant, convenience mart, or coffee shop. It's simple to eat the meal without even being completely conscious of the eating procedure (i.e. chewing, tasting, and feeling a feeling of fullness). However, on a vegetarian diet, you might need to plan meals in advance to discover foods you like and which are compliant with the eating program. Or you've may need to make careful decisions in the present time. The picking and planning procedure demands attention, concentrate, and thoughtfulness on your food choices--crucial elements of careful eating.

Wider food variety

An omnivore diet gets rid of no foods. The traditional american diet is a omnivore diet. However, most people who have a traditional diet consume a comparatively restricted variety of foods or kinds of food. For example, many conventional american dishes include beef, starch (rice or curry), and perhaps a vegetable. Dairy products are frequently utilized as side dishes, or leftovers.

On a vegetarian diet, but several conventional foods aren't compliant. Thus, when you start this diet, then you might need to find creative and experiment with meals which aren't familiar.

However, there's a caveat for this advantage. Many food makers are producing plant-based versions of standard favorites. For example, many grocery stores take vegan-friendly meatless burgers, processed poultry or turkey options, and dairy-substitutes which are created from soy along with other components. From time to time, these goods are not any fitter than their meat/dairy choice, and relying upon them can contribute to precisely the exact same restricted food palate such as a classic diet.

Potential weight reduction

Various studies have revealed that you might drop weight on a vegetarian diet. Obviously, only opting to go vegan doesn't bring about weight loss to happen. However, while you embrace this lifestyle, then you remove many foods which are high in calories and fat.

Plant-based ingestion is frequently connected with shedding weight. Back in 2018, a restricted 16-week clinical trial discovered that a vegetarian diet was shown to be outstanding to a control diet (that contained animal protein) in enhancing body fat and fat mass. And a wide evidence review printed in 2017 discovered that dietary diets are a powerful tool in the prevention and management of obesity and overweight.

Even in the event that you have problems staying

with a weight loss program, a vegetarian lifestyle could be the very best alternative. Studies also have proven that a vegetarian eating program might be more effective for weight reduction, even in the event that you don't fully adhere to the app.

Reduced food prices

Singling out a vegetarian diet can assist you to lower your food expenses. However, whether you acquire this advantage is dependent on what you consume prior to embracing this eating style and that which you opt to eat afterwards.

There's not any doubt that meat, poultry, fish, and dairy goods are costly. Some convenience foods may also be expensive. When you eliminate these foods out of the diet, then you remove the significant food prices which are connected with them.

Vegan friendly-grains and beans are often budget-friendly. And even though create and vegan-friendly convenience foods may be costly, they're most likely to cost less general than a diet full of animal-based products.

Much better for your environment

Some people select a vegetarian diet because they believe it is better for your planet. There's increased concern from the ecological community concerning the effect of livestock and livestock farming techniques in the world.

In contrast, the cultivation of vegan-friendly plants needs fewer sources (water and land) compared to creation of western foods like poultry, meat, and milk. And cows create more greenhouses gasses (methane) than crops perform, and that leads some to feel that eating beef will help to decrease the probability of global warming.
A few research studies have suggested a vegan diet is much better for the entire world compared to other diets, including the popular mediterranean diet plan.

No animal effect

Since no creatures are harmed or murdered to generate vegan-friendly foods, many select this diet due to worries regarding animal cruelty.

One study demonstrated the very popular motive for choosing a vegetarian diet would be to encourage the humane treatment of all animals. These vegans can also prevent clothing or other goods that are created from animals, fish, poultry, or even bees.

Interestingly, the next study research printed from the diary appetite discovered people who selected a vegetarian diet for moral reasons were anticipated to abide by the diet more than people who follow the plan for some other explanations.

Disadvantages

Though a vegetarian diet could be healthier for you and the entire world, this app does not work for everybody. Contemplate those drawbacks.

Restricted food options

The vegetarian diet is often known as the very restrictive variant of a diet. Surely, if you embrace this eating program, and you now eat a conventional american diet, then it is possible to expect to remove most foods out of the normal weekly menu. For many individuals, that degree of restriction is too intense.

To have a greater awareness of the scope of the limitation, bear in mind that not just are animal products removed, but any meals or merchandise which includes a creature by-product is removed. Many of the most conventional home recipes, supermarkets, and restaurant meals comprise a minumum of one creature by-product.

Obviously, lots of vegans will inform you that there's an abundance of food assortment inside this diet program. However, since it changes considerably from what you may be utilised to eating, you might discover it to be more limiting initially.

Potential nutritional deficiencies

A vegetarian diet is healthy, however there are a couple of possible nutritional supplements deficiencies which have to be dealt with. Scientists have discovered that vegetarian diets are usually lacking in calcium required for bone formation, muscle contractions, along with other essential purposes. Vegans can improve their consumption by ingestion calcium-rich foods like green leafy vegetables, legumes, sesame seeds, plus a few fruits.

Vitamin b-12, or cobalamin, is just another nutrient that might be lacking since it is found mostly in foods of animal origin. Vitamin b-12 is required for healthy nerve function and blood cell production. A deficiency may result in a condition known as pernicious anemia. While some seaweed, mushrooms, broccoli, and fermented foods can be a helpful supply of the crucial b-complex vitamin researchers have discovered that supplementation could be required for those that follow a vegetarian or vegan diet plan.

Protein might be another problem, but it is one which is readily solved. Proteins are composed of building blocks known as amino acids your body should keep muscles and organs and significant functions. Essential amino acids are the ones that your body doesn't make so that you have to get them out of the foods that you consume.

While animal fats contain all the essential amino acids plant proteins are often missing at least one of these amino acids. Thus, it's essential to eat a number of protein sources to be certain you receive all the amino acids that you want.

Vegan diets are also reduced in vitamin d, even however to be honest, are additional diets as nearly all of the vitamin d comes in exposure to sun. Two exceptional vegetarian resources of vitamin d comprise maitake mushrooms along with portobello mushrooms which were subjected to UV light. Other wise dietary supplement or nut milks can allow you to get adequate vitamin d through the wintertime.

Last, a vegetarian diet can also be deficient in just two omega-3 fatty acids known as lactic acid and lactic acid your body needs for a wholesome heart and eyes as well as mind function. But as long as you consume lots of soy, like pumpkinseeds, flaxseeds, or chia seeds, then you are going to become enough of the omega-3 fatty acid known as lipoic acid, which the body converts to another two kinds. If you are pregnant, nevertheless, it's crucial to speak with your physician to ensure to receive sufficient omega-3s throughout your pregnancy.

Demands diligence

People who follow a vegetarian diet will have to become used to carefully reading nutrition labels and ingredient lists, particularly they opt to eat foods that are processed. Foods you may presume to be liberated of creature by-products may include gelatin, whey, casein, honey, or other foods which are non-compliant to a vegetarian diet.

You will also have to carefully read nutrition labels to stay fit on a vegan diet. It's necessary to select foods that have vitamins and minerals to prevent nutrient deficiencies.

Difficulty dining outside

While searching for vegan-friendly meals, customers can read merchandise information. But should you eat someone's house or in a restaurant, then you do not have access to a ingredient listing. Because of this, dining out can be challenging for people who pick a vegetarian diet.

A couple of restaurants make a notice of vegetarian or vegan foods in their menus, but not a lot. You may have the ability to create a vegetarian meal in the side or salads dishes they serve. But you will need to ask to be certain that no animal products are employed in the groundwork.

And from time to time, even inquiring about food is not valuable. It is not unusual for well-meaning restaurant employees (or well-intentioned family and friends) to presume that healthful foods are vegetarian if they do not contain milk. But that is not always the situation. Vegetable soup, as an instance, could be produced with broth which utilized a creature bone such as flavoring.

Many vegetarian specialists advocate that when dining in someone's home, deliver a recipe which you are able to enjoy and you can share with other people. And select restaurants that you understand to become vegan-savvy.

Unrealistic expectations

While consuming a vegetarian diet is very likely to make health benefits and also a fitter weight, it isn't a guarantee. By way of instance, if you're attempting to slim down, then you still have to be conscious of the foods that you select and the amount you consume.

There's an growing quantity of processed foods. Lots of times, these foods are only too unhealthy--comprising more calories and fat as their conventional counterparts.

And health benefits aren't a slam dunk either. A study printed in the journal of the american college of cardiology compared a high number of girls who ate a healthful vegetarian diet (like whole grains, vegetables, fruits, nuts, beans, oils, tea and coffee) to people who ate a much less wholesome vegan meals (like juices, sweetened drinks, processed grains, grains, fries(and candies). Researchers reasoned that the fitter vegan diet led to a considerably lower risk for cardiovascular disorder, whereas the healthy vegetarian diet has been associated with a greater risk.

Social isolation

People's food options frequently come under scrutiny by family, friends, colleagues, and other acquaintances. You could realize that you're contested and contested about your motives for choosing this particular lifestyle. In addition, people who don't understand how to adapt your daily diet can exclude you in social gatherings. Or worse, that they can invite you and invite you to consume foods which aren't vegan-friendly.

Some vegetarian sites address these problems and supply advice for all those adapting to the eating mode. Experts recommend that you just reach out into other vegans in your area and build up a community, while being patient with people who don't know your options.

CHAPTER SIX

VEGAN DIET VS. OTHER DIETS: WHICH IS BEST?

Vegan diets have grown in popularity in the past few decades. Actually, a few sources have reported that a 600 percent gain in the number of individuals identifying as dinner involving 2014 and 2017.

The availability of vegetarian foods at mainstream supermarket shops, vegan menu options at restaurants, and press reports reporting wellness advantages of vegetarian diets have led to this tendency.

Nevertheless, the vegetarian diet is not right for everybody. Some specialists say that the diet is difficult to keep and many others have mentioned concerns regarding the deficiency of certain nutrients within this strategy. If you're thinking about a vegan way of life, see the way the eating strategy contrasts with other similar diets prior to making your choice.

Usda tips

It can be difficult to compare a vegetarian diet to usda guidelines --or into some diet for that matter-- since there's not any"standard" vegetarian diet. Unlike some diet programs for weight loss or improved health, there's not any particular macronutrient condition, calorie rule, or foods that are required.

Rather, the vegetarian diet only requires that you prevent calcium-rich products, such as beef, poultry, poultry, milk, eggs, and also (in some instances) honey.) Because of this, there might be significant nutritional variation from a vegetarian diet into another.

Yet, a few studies have assessed vegetarian eating routines and also have been able to present certain generalizations regarding the nutrient and food consumption to a typical vegetarian diet. With the assumptions, the vegetarian diet could be contrasted to usda guidelines along with other diets.

Present usda nutrition guidelines imply we eat foods

such as veggies, vegetables, fruit, low-carb or low-fat legumes, protein, and oils. The guidelines also indicate that americans limit saturated fats and trans fats fats, added sugars, and sodium.

On a vegetarian diet, you might eat foods in all of those suggested meals groups. Various studies have revealed that vegetarian eaters typically eat more vegetables, fruits, and wholesome oils compared to individuals that follow with a non-vegan diet.3 but, there's absolutely not any dairy intake on a vegetarian diet. Milk options (for instance, nut-based"milk" goods) are regarded as a protein as opposed to a dairy product at nutritional tests.

You're also prone to naturally restrict foods according to usda guidelines. As an instance, the majority of the saturated fat absorbed at a conventional american diet comes from dairy and meat products. These foods aren't consumed on a vegetarian diet. Furthermore, many vegetarian eaters additionally prevent processed foods to health reasons or because they comprise animal by-products as components. Processed processed foods often contain added sugars and surplus sodium. And a few processed foods contain trans fats.

Nutrients

Nutrient intake might be tricky for a few on a vegetarian diet. Especially, a number of studies have proven that calcium, protein, and vitamin b12 consumption is reduced when after this eating mode. Additionally, vegetarian diets might also be reduced in potassium, iron, and vitamin d.

Calcium

Usda guidelines imply that we have 1,000 to 1,200 mg of calcium daily. For a lot of individuals, consuming milk products helps them fulfill that objective. However, because you don't eat milk on a vegetarian diet, you need to get calcium from other sources (for example, kale, pinto beans, or fortified orange juice). One study noted that a standard vegan eater absorbs closer to 738 mg of calcium every day.

Vitamin b12

Your vitamin b12 consumption might be reduced on

a vegetarian diet. Vitamin b12 helps regulate metabolism and can be found chiefly in animal and fish products. The usda recommends that adults eat 2.4 micrograms (mcg) of b12 every day. According to the american academy of nutrition and dietetics, vegans should regularly consume dependable sources of b12--significance fortified foods or b-12 comprising nutritional supplements or else they might eventually become deficient, as revealed in the case studies of vegan babies, kids, and adults.

Protein

Protein could be another issue for many, but the american academy of nutrition and dietetics says that individuals following vegetarian diets normally meet or surpass protein recommendations, given caloric intakes are sufficient. There are many vegan-friendly protein resources, including tofu, seeds, nuts, legumes, and grains.

Usda guidelines suggest that adults have 10% to 35 percent of the total calories every day in the protein. Various studies assessing vegetarian diets also have discovered an intake of 13 percent to 14 percent from protein is more average. Although it's still lower than the number generally consumed with a non-vegan, the quote remains within recommended guidelines.

Iron

As soon as we think about iron-rich foods, beef usually springs to mind. But, there are lots of vegan resources of iron, such as, legumes and legumes, cashews, potatoes, and green leafy vegetables such as spinach. If you're worried about your iron intake, then pairing iron-rich foods with meals high in vitamin c may boost iron absorption.

Iodine

Plant-based diets may be high in iodine. Vegans who don't consume iodized salt or sea vegetables might be at risk of nutrient deficiency. In the event you use sea salt, then check to find out whether it's additional iodine.

Vitamin d

Low vitamin d intakes have been reported in several vegetarians and vegans, as well as non serum or plasma 25-hydroxyvitamin d amounts. Ever since your body also produces vitamin d in sun, very low vitamin d intake could be an issue in winter months and early spring, particularly for people residing at higher latitudes.

Calories

A vegetarian diet doesn't limit your caloric consumption. There's no reason to count calories on a vegetarian diet unless your objective is to drop weight. Even after that, you might be able to lose weight by simply reducing serving sizes and picking nutrient-rich, lower-calorie meals. However, you might not have to.

Studies show that these subsequent vegetarian diets obviously consume fewer calories than those after different diets. Actually, studies have revealed that even in the event that you don't adhere to a vegetarian diet absolutely, you're very likely to eat fewer calories and lose more fat than you would to a vegetarian diet, pesco-vegetarian, semi-vegetarian, or omnivore diet plan.

But you might want to make sure you're getting sufficient energy in the event you change into a vegetarian diet. To gauge your overall calorie requirements for daily, you may use a nutritional supplement. This calculator protects your age, sex, aims, and action level into consideration to ascertain the ideal amount for you.

You may believe a vegetarian diet is much more restrictive than a traditional American diet also referred to as an omnivore diet. In the end, a lot of individuals who change into the eating fashion need to remove a lot of their preferred foods out of their diet program. But going vegan can motivate you to consume a broader range of meals.

Without meat onto your plate at mealtime, then you might be motivated to attempt processed grains or soy-based carbohydrates, such as tofu, tempeh, or edamame. And because vegetables will probably play a larger part in your everyday diet, you might choose to try new kinds. Searching for seasonal fruits and vegetables can allow you to relish the yummiest choices at a reduce cost.

However, the rising prevalence of vegan-friendly processed foods might lead some to consume a vegetarian diet with less number and diminished nutrition. Plant-based processed, processed, other foods (such as meatless burgers or vegan-friendly microwave dishes) provide little in the way of excellent nutrition and make it a lot easier for some to remain in a restricted food rut.

Similar bites

The diets similar to a vegetarian diet are additional plant-friendly eating programs . Not all those plans entirely eradicates beef, but every one depends heavily on foods that are fermented. Scientists have compared the vegetarian diet to a vegetarian diet plan, a vegetarian flexitarian dietplan, a pescatarian diet plan, as well as also an omnivore diet plan (no meals excluded) and reasoned that a vegetarian diet is the most healthful. The results, according to evaluation scales, also revealed vegans had the lowest calcium intakes

A vegetarian diet is somewhat like a vegetarian diet because meat and fish (like red meat, white meat, fish or fowl) isn't consumed. Most drinkers eat eggs and milk (lacto-ovo drinkers), however a few prevent dairy and eat eggs (ovo vegetarians). Lacto-vegetarians prevent eggs but eat milk.

General nourishment: when investigators compared a standard vegetarian diet to a vegetarian diet working with a healthy eating index (which assesses how foods compare to recommended directions) that the vegetarian diet plan scored lower than a vegetarian diet but still comparatively large. Protein, calcium, and vitamin intake can be greater with this strategy because dairy eggs and foods may be consumed.

Health advantages: a vegetarian diet is associated with several of exactly the identical health advantages as a vegetarian diet, such as a decrease risk of cardiovascular disease, diabetes, and hypertension.

Weight reduction: because removing meat and animal-based products helps cut calories and fat from the daily diet, a vegetarian diet is very likely to be successful for weight reduction, according to a number of studies. But because wholesome processed foods are getting more common, it's still feasible to overeat on a vegetarian diet plan although it is not as inclined than on a conventional diet.

Sustainability: as a vegetarian diet may be easier to adhere to than a vegetarian diet, a few still find it tricky to keep. But several vegetarian specialists advise that you try a vegetarian diet plan prior to going into a vegetarian diet due to the addition of milk and egg products helps many people today feel fuller and revel in conventional foods. If losing weight is your goal, sustainability might not matter. Studies have discovered that adherence rates do not change considerably between vegetarian, vegan, flexitarian, pescetarian, and omnivore diets to fat reduction.

But on a flexitarian diet , you consume mostly based on vegetarian guidelines. But, those who recognize as flexitarian sometimes eat meat and fish.

General nourishment: portion of this flexitarian diet

to the vegetarian diet utilizing the healthy eating index discovered this type of vegetarian eating might be somewhat more healthy than the vegetarian diet, however fitter than a vegetarian diet. The occasional addition of seafood and meat may help a few with this diet to raise their protein and vitamin b12 consumption.

Health advantages: as a flexitarian diet plan is primarily a vegetarian diet, people that follow this eating fashion are more very likely to obtain the very same advantages, such as improved cardiovascular health and a reduced risk for several chronic ailments.

Weight reduction: eating a typical meat or fish meal is not very likely to modify the calorie consumption of a vegetarian diet to ensure it is less effective when weight reduction is your objective. Because of this, flexitarian diets are more inclined to be equally as powerful once you're attempting to eliminate weight. Occasional meat-based meals might even help a stick for their diet more.

Sustainability: even though studies have found

small variation between healthful diets (such as this one) as it has to do with adherence, most experts indicate that a flexitarian diet is significantly more sustainable just because it allows for occasional indulgences. Traveling, eating outside, and interacting with friends is very likely to be simpler with this strategy.

Pescatarian

Should you follow a more pescetarian diet, you consume mostly plant-based foods however contain fish in your diet too.

General nourishment: employing the healthy eating index, researchers believed the pescetarian diet reduced compared to vegetarian diet program but nearly the exact same as the vegetarian and vegetarian flexitarian dietplan. But when utilizing a distinct healthier eating scale dependent on the mediterranean diet plan, this eating mode scored greater than the vegetarian diet plan and flexitarian diet plan (but still lower compared to a vegetarian diet). The focus on fish intake can help to boost not just your protein consumption but your consumption of healthy carbohydrates, such as omega-3 fatty acids.)

Health advantages: you are most likely to get the identical wellbeing advantages with this diet because you want a vegetarian or vegan diet but you could like a couple more in case you eat fish which are high in omega-3 fatty acids. These fatty acids help to keep healthy blood vessels, reduce ldl cholesterol and reduce both cholesterol levels and blood pressure.

Weight reduction: when compared with some traditional american diet plan, this eating strategy is very likely to be effective for weight reduction. When compared with vegetarian and vegan programs, it's very likely to be equally as powerful. The usage of fish may improve your calorie consumption slightly (based on the kind you select) but you might also raise satiety and adherence.

Sustainability: if you're currently a normal fish eater, then this diet is very likely to be sustainable. However, for others, it might be less . Not everybody is comfortable cooking fish on a normal basis and fish (that can be much more healthy than breaded or processed fish) could be costly and more difficult to locate.

Mediterranean

A mediterranean diet contains food groups recommended by the usda. Animal products are absorbed, but structurally. The focus is really on veggies, grains, seeds, nuts, and plant-based wholesome oils.

General nourishment: this nutritional supplement is much more likely compared to vegetarian diet to align with nutrient guidelines offered from the usda. Foods that are high in saturated fat (meat and dairy) are reduced and foods that promote wellbeing (whole grains, veggies) are invited . But because animal milk and products are still absorbed in tiny amounts, protein, calcium, and vitamin amounts are not as inclined to be endangered.

Health advantages: the Mediterranean diet was broadly researched and is connected with a vast assortment of health advantages including a lower chance of cardiovascular disease, cancer, and other chronic ailments.

Weight reduction: most researchers have assessed the mediterranean diet's efficacy in regards to losing weight. Many have discovered the eating plan to work for weight reduction (as powerful as similar low-carb diets) and many others have discovered that although it might not promote weight reduction significantly, it can help prevent weight gain with time.

Sustainability: the mediterranean diet might be the most sustainable diet in comparison to some other rigorous dietary diets, like the vegetarian diet and the vegetarian diet plan. No meals are off-limits with this strategy. Instead, wholesome foods are highlighted and not as wholesome foods are lessened.

CHAPTER SEVEN

GETTING STARTED WITH A VEGAN DIET

A vegetarian diet is one where no creature foods or creature by-products have been consumed. A vegetarian diet includes vegetables, fruits, grains, seeds, nuts, and soy products, but no meat, poultry, fish, milk, eggs, or honey.

If you currently follow with an omnivore eating fashion (minimal dietary limitations), moving straight to a more restrictive eating strategy such as the vegetarian diet can be complicated. Because of this, many nutrition experts indicate a slow strategy.

By way of example, some people today find victory on a vegetarian diet by embracing a flexitarian diet first. A flexitarian diet really is a modified vegetarian diet which lets you consume meat on a few restricted events. As soon as you're familiar with all the flexitarian eating mode, it is possible to completely embrace a vegetarian diet then eventually go vegan.

Another approach that might help ease the transition would be that the "add, subtract later" strategy. In accordance with the process, you begin to add pleasing vegetarian dishes into your own menu prior to subtracting foods which are non-compliant. You remove the foods you're dependent on last--if your own vegan eating strategy has a solid basis.

Irrespective of which approach you choose, remember to give your time first embracing this dietary plan. A vegetarian diet may provide many health benefits, however based on where you start from, it might take months, weeks, or even more time to find out how to store, cook, and also completely appreciate vegetarian eating.

Your own calorie goals

Studies show that people who follow a vegetarian diet generally consume fewer calories than people who consume other kinds of diets. This calorie loss generally occurs naturally since foods which are removed on a vegetarian diet are foods which are far high in calories and fat, such as dairy and meat. Because of this, you might gain from weight reduction when changing to the eating style.

However, if you're already at a wholesome weight when you move vegan, then you will want to be certain you eat enough calories every day to keep wellness. Consuming a lot of calories may result in diminished vitality, a reduction of muscular mass, along with other issues.

And, of course, consuming a lot of calories may lead to weight gain--no matter of the diet plan you select. Though vegetarian diets are normally lower in calories, even should you assemble meals around foods which are full of fat and surplus sugar it's still feasible to lose weight. So, on a vegetarian diet, then you need to be certain you keep the appropriate energy equilibrium.

The amount of calories (energy) that you want each day is dependent upon a number of factors, such as weight, height, and activity level. Your aims seeing weight reduction or weight reduction will also be significant. Calculators such as the one below will offer a personalized estimate of the amount of calories that you want.

Should you typically construct your meals about a serving of beef, eggs, fish, or poultry (and you would like to keep your present weight), it can be of help to observe how you could replace these calories using vegan-friendly alternatives.

- A three-ounce serving of meat comprises about 180 calories. A vegan-friendly veggie beans may provide 130-175 calories.

- A three-ounce serving of salmon comprises about 180 calories. A one-cup dose of lentils supplies approximately 220 calories.

- A three-ounce functioning of chicken breast feeding comprises about 102 calories. A five-ounce dose of kale supplies approximately 100 calories.

- 2 scrambled eggs supply approximately comprises about 150 calories. 1 cup of cooked yogurt supplies approximately 166 calories.

When you're searching for ways to enjoy vegetarian protein resources, recall that you're able to raise your calorie consumption by utilizing healthy fats at the preparation of the meals. Moderate quantities of vitamins that are fermented, such as olive oil, coconut oil, or flaxseed oil supply polyunsaturated and monounsaturated fats which may help boost cardiovascular health.

Hydration tips

Staying hydrated is comparatively simple on a vegetarian diet.

Fruits and berries

Should you increase your fruit and vegetable consumption on a vegetarian diet (as most men and women do) it could be a lot easier to remain hydrated daily. Scientific studies have revealed that increasing your vegetable and fruit consumption may encourage a healthy water balance within your system.

Water constitutes almost 90 percent of the burden of fruits and vegetables that we eat.

Boost daily hydration by swallowing melonfruits, vegetables, and citrus fruits. Vegetables which improve hydration include cabbage, broccoli, cauliflower, celery, cucumber, and lots of more.

Dairy alternatives

Dairy products (such as milk and yogurt-based drinks) aren't compliant. But, nut"milks" might be a suitable alternative if you're utilized to preparing or drinking foods using milk. Most grocery stores take milk choices like cashew milk, almond milk, almond milk, and lots of more.

Remember, however, the fda is considering laws to eliminate the title"milk" from non-meat choices.4 thus, once you're searching for these products, you might have to read labels carefully when making your choice. Additionally, remember that some products might contain non-vegan components, including whey protein isolate or casein.

Other drinks

The majority of other drinks are vegan-friendly. By way of example, tea, many lemonade, fruit juice, and coffee is generally free of milk or creature by-products. But, there are a couple notable exceptions.

Drinks flavored with honey are usually prevented on a vegetarian diet. Not all vegans avoid soda, but should you decide to, then you are going to have to read drink labels carefully to make certain your beverage is more compliant.

Additionally, broth-based drinks are usually not vegan-friendly since they're frequently created out of bones of a creature.

Grocery staples

Changing to a vegetarian diet can provide you an opportunity to explore unique areas of the grocery shop. Perhaps you will opt to think about a new sort of marketplace, like a farmer's market, or even health food shop.

Consider these nutritious choices located in various sections. Remember that purchasing in volume and picking seasonal create can help keep your budget on track.

Bulk foods

From the majority foods place, you can save money by buying only the amount that you want. These meals are usually more affordable because packing costs are removed.

- Flax, chia, hemp, sesame, or citrus seeds

- Quinoa, farro, bulgur, barley, oats, along with whole grains

- Almonds, cashews, pistachios, and other tree nuts

- Peanuts along with other beans

- Citrus fruit including calcium-rich dried figs

Create section

Pick fruits and vegetables that provide the minerals and vitamins which are likely to reduce when eliminating meat and milk out of your diet plan. Choose calcium-rich veggies and fruits like kale, figs. And protein-rich create, such as spinach, can help you keep muscle mass.

Mushrooms are just another food to put in on at the aisle. If you're having difficulty removing beef out of your foods, mushrooms supply a salty, meaty alternate.

Other healthy fruits and veggies to consider include:

spicy peppers

mustard or collard greens

arugula, swiss chard, and other leafy greens

bok choy

okra

asparagus

cabbage

eggplant

spaghetti skillet

oranges

apples

avocado

tomato

fiber-rich berries such as sweet

Frozen foods

Many grocery stores sell vegan convenience foods, such as microwavable meals, frozen meat replacements, and other fast fast-food design offerings. Bear in mind that although those foods are compliant in your vegan eating program, they do not necessarily offer decent nutrition.

Rather, think about stocking up on processed frozen foods such as

frozen noodle (edamame)

frozen berry

frozen veggies

coconut or nut-based ice-cream

Cereals, canned, and dry goods

At the midst aisles of the supermarket, you'll discover many nutritious vegan-friendly offerings, such as beans and fortified cereal. While buying beans, look at buying the dried variety instead of canned products. Some canned products are high in sodium.

white legumes

kidney beans

dark beans

whole-grain cereal

dried spices and herbs

rolled oats

tahini

plant-based oils

whole-grain crackers

spicy peppers like bean soup or curry soup

protein powder made using rice, soy, or pea protein

Refrigerated section

You may be used to picking dairy products such as milk and cheese in this segment. But if you look beyond the products you'll come across products which are tasty and compliant with your own diet. Start looking for

soy milk (calcium-fortified)

noodle berry

coconut milk

plant-based yogurt (like coconut milk)

orange juice, fortified with calcium

tempeh or tofu

hummus

kombucha

spicy foods like sauerkraut or miso paste

Recipe ideas

Learning how to cook new foods may make adapting into the vegetarian diet simpler. Put money into a cookbook, locate recipes that are online, or research a vegetarian meal program to receive a feeling of several distinct tactics to enjoy fruits, veggies, grains, seeds, beans, and wholesome oils.

Breakfast

Begin your day with meals which offer protein and fiber that will help you feel complete through feverish morning actions.

Low-sugar coconut raspberry oatmeal

Complete time: 20 minutes

Prep time: 5 minutes

Cook time: 15 minutes

Servings: 1

Nutrition highlights (per serving)

223 calories

8g fat

33g carbohydrates

5g protein

Packed with filling fiber , oatmeal is the best method to fuel the beginning of your day using long-term energy. That pretty in pink bowl of coconut cherry oatmeal is obviously garnished with suspended raspberries, therefore it includes no extra sugar. Additionally, it's simple to create for busy morningsjust sew every thing together until creamy and function!

Ingredient

1/4 cup steel cut oats, raw

3/4 cup almond milk

1/2 cup frozen desserts

 pinch of salt

1 tbsp unsweetened coconut batter

1 tsp chia seeds

Preparation

1. In a little kettle, whisk with yogurt, almond nuts, milk, and salt on medium heat.

2. Simmer 10 to 20 minutes, stirring occasionally to

avoid burning, until ginger are tender and creamy. In the event the oats are receiving too dry, then add 1/4 cup water into the kettle.

3. Pour oatmeal into a bowl and top with coconut scents and chia.

Fixing variations and substitutions

Simmering oats using frozen fruit really is a special method. Not only will it add flavorful sweet taste, but in addition, it sweetens the oatmeal without including sugar. Additionally, it turns out your breakfast a gorgeous shade of colour! The podcasts i utilized in this recipe would be my favorite since they divide to the oatmeal, however in addition, this is tasty with frozen cherries, berries, blueberries, and strawberry too.

When these oats receive a hint of sweetness in the naturally occurring sugars in fruit, even should you want your oats somewhat sweeter, then stir in a teaspoon or two of honey, pure maple syrup, or your own treasured non-caloric sweetener.

Getting tired of oatmeal? Consider experimenting

with additional whole grains for dinner! Alter the oats for 1/2 cup cooked quinoa, farro, or barley to relish unique textures. Quinoa is much more porridge-like feel when utilized in coconut milk, even whilst farro and barley are far bigger grains with much more of a texture.

Cooking and serving tips

If you end up always in a hurry in the morning, make a large batch of the oatmeal and shop individual containers in the refrigerator. You will only wish to bring a bit more coconut milk to cut it out until reheating in the microwave.

I recommend my customers, particularly those with diabetes, comprise food which includes fat and protein . Both require more time to digest than carbohydrate, helping keep blood glucose stable before your next snack or meal.

Additionally, it can help keep you fuller longer. To include fat and protein into this recipe, combine this oatmeal sprinkled along with your selection of nuts or using a egg or two over the other side. You might also stir into a spoonful of protein powder. Just be certain you select one without additional sugar and also add a little additional liquid to keep it from drying out.

Healthy fruit salad with citrus mint dressing
Complete time: 10 minutes

Prep time: 10 minutes

Cook time: 0 minute

Servings: 4 (1/2 cup per day)

Nutrition highlights (per serving)

58 calories

0g fat

15g carbohydrates

1g protein

Go natural once you're seeking to satisfy your teeth. This simple fruit salad brings together the flavors of your favourite fruit. The mint and citrus dressing table, made of freshly squeezed oranges and limes, ties the whole dish together. What additional dinner may supply you with just as much vitamin fiber, antioxidants, and also no-sugar added goodness?

Ingredients

two clementine's, peeled and every slice cut in to 3 bits

1/2 cup fresh berries, diced

1/4 cup berries, sliced in half

1/2 cup oranges, diced

1/2 cup pineapple, diced

juice of 1 lemon

juice of 1 tsp

20 mint leaves chopped

Preparation

1. Mix all components in a big bowl. Chill before serving.

Fixing variations and substitutions

This recipe does not have any guidelines --you can swap in all fruit at equivalent quantities. Utilize your preferred or use leftover fruit up in your refrigerator. Each fruit provides its profile of special antioxidants and tastes. You will not be selling yourself short on nourishment if you exchange any outside.

Cooking and serving tips

This fruit salad is served fresh and cold. If you will not be working out the entire batch, look at earning less omit leftovers.

It is up to you if you would like to depart the lean clementine skin before mixing with fruit. Peeling the individual sections is time intensive, and therefore don't be concerned about leaving the person skins.

Chia pudding with honeydew melon

Cook time: 240 minutes

 Complete time: 245 minutes

Prep time: 5 minutes

Servings: two

Nutrition highlights (per serving)

207 calories

11g fat

22g carbohydrates

8g protein

Tiny chia seeds are not only for houseplants. This small superfood packs in large quantities of nutrients, such as inflammation battling omega-3 fats.

When saturated in liquid, chia seeds gel, developing a creamy and thick pudding that stays saturated in fat and is also excellent for people experiencing heartburn. Adhering to a lower-fat diet might help prevent reflux and heartburn. In addition, this velvety mix feels like a guilty pleasure but can be really a wholesome indulgence. This recipe also includes 10 g of hunger-fighting fiber daily that is 40 percent of their daily recommendation!

Ingredients

1 cup vanilla soy milk

1/4 cup chia seeds

1/2 cup finely chopped honeydew melon

Preparation

1. Blend soy milk and chia seeds in a bowl and combine well.

2. Cover with plastic wrap and move to the fridge. Let me set for two hours.

3. After 2 hours mix gently and come back to the refrigerator to cool for two more hours or up to overnight.

4. Top with melon prior to serving.

Fixing variations and substitutions

This recipe works well with any kind of milk or milk substitute. Soy milk is a much greater protein choice, however, almond milk is just another low-fat alternative.

Drink this pudding as dinner, breakfast, or even a late night snack topped with. Any kind of fruit. If you produce a batch of chia pudding, then you can top it using distinct fruit during the week to get variety. Most fruit are heartburn-friendly. Green apples, however, might cause heartburn in certain.

To get a little additional crunch, sprinkle a tablespoon of granola just prior to serving. Be smart in adding longer, as granola may acquire calorie-dense.

Cooking and serving tips

Shop ready pudding covered with plastic wrap in the fridge for up to two weeks. When saving for longer intervals, cover with plastic wrap so the wrapping is in contact with all your pudding. This may stop a skin from forming across the surface of it.

Steak and dinner

Replace meat-based foods with heavy, hot dishes created with savory veggies

Shredded brussels sprouts and roasted lentil salad

Complete time: 35 minutes

Prep time: 10 minutes

Cook time: 25 minutes

Servings: 4 (1/2 cup per day)

Nutrition highlights (per serving)

137 calories

5g fat

19g carbohydrates

7g protein

Lentils and brussels sprouts discuss the spotlight in this shredded brussels sprouts and roasted lentil salad.

Like many beans , lentils are an affordable and sustainable supply of nourishment --you can purchase a pound for just 2 bucks and take in a lot of filling protein and fiber per serving. Additionally, they supply blood-pressure controlling potassium, blood-health encouraging iron, without any fat. That is a winning combination for a daily diet useful in managing hypertension.

When roasted and paired with crispy brussels

sprouts, then you've got a winning meatless dinner or a foundation for extra protein, such as poultry or even fish.

Ingredients

1/2 cup cooked legumes

1 medium carrot

1/2 red bell pepper

1/2 tsp kosher salt

1 tbsp olive oil

4 big brussels sprouts, stained

8 tsp, chopped

2 tbsp lemon juice

1/4 teaspoon ground black pepper

Preparation

1. Line a large baking sheet and preheat the oven to 350f.

2. Toss the peas, carrot, and bell pepper and olive oil and arrange on the baking sheet. Roast for 20 to

25, assessing stirring and on everything about halfway .

3. When prepared, slice the lettuce into thin rounds and then dice the bell pepper.

4. Blend lentils, vegetables, stained brussels sprouts, olives, lemon juice, and black pepper.

Fixing variations and substitutions

It is possible to use any colour bell pepper along with any type of olives you've got handy.

In regards to olives, you'll detect a number of kinds in the shop --manzanilla and kalamata are just two of the very prevalent ones. Green olives (such as manzanilla) and black olives (such as kalamatas) vary in their ripeness, using dark olives being riper than green ones. Their nourishment content is almost identical--both provide healthful monounsaturated fats as well as a few minerals.however, keep a watch out for the sodium. It is going to change based on the sort of brine utilized, so have a moment to compare labels.

Additionally, you do not desire stuffed olives with

this particular recipe, simply ones that are striped, but notice that green buds are often full of pimientos, garlic, almonds, and other add-ins, that will impact their caloric counts.

Cooking and serving tips

When you've got lots of brussels sprouts you can fix them at a food processor. Since we are just using four, simply use a knife. Cut each sprout in half an hour, and then, holding on the challenging stem finish, finely slice it till you arrive at the end. It's possible to discard the difficult end.

Triple tomato pasta with spinach and white beans

Entire time: 30 minutes

Prep time: 10 min

Cook time: 20 min

Servings: 4

Tomatoes get their red color from lycopene, an antioxidant which may help to avoid cancer and cardiovascular disease. Cooking berries actually can help increase lycopene content, hence possibly fostering its high-value power.

Along with lycopene this recipe provides great nutrient advantages in your cannellini beans. These legumes are packed with fiber, at 6 g a half cup serving. They're also among the maximum potassium beans on the market, a micronutrient and electrolyte that could help reduce blood pressure.

Ingredients

8 oz whole wheat penne pasta

1 can low sodium cannellini beans

1 tbsp olive oil

1 pack baby lettuce

2 cups cherry tomatoes, diced

1 cup sun-dried berries in petroleum

1/4 cup sliced/slivered tsp

1 tbsp tomato paste

1 tsp balsamic vinegar

2 tsp garlic (or 1 teaspoon minced)

2 tsp dried peppermint

1/2 tsp salt

1/4 tsp black pepper

1/4 tsp crushed red pepper

Preparation

1. Cook pasta according to package instructions.

2. Blend pesto components (slivered almonds through crushed red pepper) in a food processor and mix until mostly smooth; a few tiny chunks are fine. You might want to some clutter water to lean, but don't include more than a couple tbsp because the sauce is intended to be thick.

3. Drain and wash cannellini beans.

4. Insert olive oil into a bowl and heat to medium. Insert baby spinach and cook until wilted. Remove from heat.

5. Blend the legumes, spinach, and berries into a big pot. Add the pesto and blend well.

6. Split right into four bowls and serve.

Fixing variations and substitutions

If you can't find sun-dried berries in the oil, then you can substitute 3/4 cup bagged sun-dried berries using 1/4 cup olive oil. It works better if berries are soaked from the oil for an hour.

Cooking and serving tips

Leftover pesto tastes yummy as a sandwich spread. Additionally, it freezes well.

Dark bean-arugula tostadas with turmeric guacamole

Complete time: 20 minutes

Prep time: 10 minutes

Cook time: 10 minutes

Servings: two (two tostadas each)

Nutrition highlights (per serving)

461 calories

14g fat

70g carbs

19g protein

Eating more fermented foods might help boost your intake of antioxidants, including fiber, and minerals and vitamins. Following is a tasty, meatless model of a mexican classic.

These tacos contain black legumes , that have elevated levels of a powerful antioxidant known as anthocyanins, as a result of their own darkly pigmented skins. That is where the anti inflammatory, antioxidant benefits finish --that the turmeric from the guacamole is also a potent antioxidant. Additionally, the legumes contribute fiber and also iron whereas the avocado provides healthy low-fat . This protein-fat combo keeps you awake more --considerably more than it will require you to whip this recipe up.

Ingredients

4 6-inch entire grain corn tortillas

1.5 tsp olive oil

2 cups canned black beans, rinsed and drained

1/2 cup supper

1/2 medium avocado, peeled and diced

1 tbsp finely chopped red onion

1 medium clove garlic

1 tsp fresh lemon juice

1/4 tsp powdered turmeric

1/4 teaspoon ground cumin

1/8 tsp salt

pinch of ground black pepper

4 cups arugula

1/2 cup sliced tomato

1/4 tsp red pepper flakes (optional)

Preparation

1. Preheat the oven to 350f.
2. Brush 2 teaspoon of olive oil on each side of each tortilla, put onto a baking sheet, and bake until crispy, about 10 seconds.

3. In a blender, pulse legumes and cauliflower until roughly half the beans are pureed and half stay chunky. Add water1 tbsp at a time, should you want to narrow the mix. If you would rather the legumes warm rather than room temperature, then warmth at a microwave-safe dish 1 minute, or till heated through.

4. In a medium bowl, mix the avocado, red onion, garlic, lemon juice, garlic, cumin, salt, and pepper together until smooth.

5. Heating 2 tbsp of water in a big pan and then add the four cups of arugula, mixing until just slightly wilted, then eliminate water.

6. Build your own tostada. Distribute the salsa and bean mix on the chopped tortilla and top with all the wilted arugula, chopped celery, guacamole, and drizzle of red pepper .

Fixing variations and substitutions

If you are not a fan of just don't possess black beans useful, use pinto beans or kidney beans rather. Or, try out a variant with garbanzo beans and utilize curry powder at the guacamole instead of peppermint and peppermint. You will still get the filling iron, fiber, and antioxidants.

Brand new sprouts, such as sunflower sprouts, can substitute the arugula if you want a crunchier, raw topping. In reality, you may use spinach or kale rather than the arugula in case you are not fond of the flavor.

Wish to create this dish a burrito bowl? Change the tortilla outside for cooked quinoa or brown rice. Substitute lime for lemon to bring a somewhat different taste profile and swap from chili powder instead of cumin to put in a gentle twist.

Cooking and serving tips

Allow the garlic sit 10 minutes once you mince it and the human body will consume a lot of the antioxidant compounds that are active.

Corn tortilla freeze nicely and thaw fast, so keep extras from the freezer in the event you do not intend to utilize them inside a week.

You can inform a avocado is ripe if it is stem falls

easily off and leaves a patch of vivid green flesh vulnerable.

If you prefer milder tortillas, brush with oil and heat in a skillet till only warm.

Snacks

Use snack time as a excuse to enhance your fiber or protein consumption.

Versatile glazed edamame recipe

Complete time: 5 minutes

Prep time: 5 minutes

Cook time: 0 minute

Servings: 5 (1/2 cup per day)

Nutrition highlights (per serving)

121 calories

7g fat

9g carbohydrates

8g protein

Immature soybeans, selected and functioned green, have been known as edamame. They've been appreciated for several years in japan, korea, china, and hawaii, and so are currently easily accessible u.s. grocery shops, at the frozen food department.

Edamame is generally eaten as finger foods and may be served as a party snack or after college. Decide on the edamame up from the stem end, place the entire thing in your mouth, then suck the beans out, and then discard the pods.

Ingredients

12 ounce frozen edamame pods

1 tbsp toasted sesame oil

1 tsp hot lavender oil

1 tbsp peeled, grated ginger root

1 tablespoon reduced sodium soy sauce

1 tbsp rice vinegar

1 tablespoon packed light brown sugar

1/4 tsp crushed red pepper flakes

Preparation

1. In a large saucepan, bring two quarts of water to a boil. Insert the frozen edamame and then return the kettle to a boil. Reduce the heat and simmer for a minute. Pouring from yourself to avert the warm steam drain the edamame pods into a colander and rinse with cold water to halt the cooking.

2. In a huge skillet over medium-high warmth, warm the oil. Add the ginger and sauté, stirring often, for 1 to 2 minutes, before the ginger begins to brown. Add the soy sauce, ginger, and brown sugar and stir till the sugar has been dissolved. Add the edamame. Reduce heat to moderate and stir with a silicone spatula till the sauce caramelizes and decreases to create a sip over the edamame pods. Scrape the sauce away from the sides and bottom of the skillet occasionally throughout the caramelization procedure. Sprinkle with red pepper flakes, if desired, and serve hot.

Variations and substitutions

Limit the proportions of toasted to hot eucalyptus

oil to suit your palate.

To make this recipe fermented, utilize fermented soy sauce or fermented tamari.

Cooking and serving tips

Do not rely on the boiling water. If you do not utilize enough water to cook the edamame pods, so it is going to take too much time to go back to a boil, so the time will be away, along with the pods will be emptied by the time they've boiled for 1 second.

Fresh ginger and citrus oil are low fodmap kitchen key weapons. Little bottles of sesame oil can be found at all grocery stores. Read the label closely. "plain" sesame oil could possibly be called toasted; it's a dark brownish color. Spicy sesame oil is more red in colour and can be, as marketed, sexy stuff. A bit goes a very long way, therefore keep sesame oil from the fridge after opening so it is going to remain fresh between applications.

Cumin-lime roasted chickpeas recipe

Complete time: 45 minutes

Prep time: 5 minutes

Cook time: 40 minutes

Servings: 3 (1/4 cup per day)

Nutrition highlights (per serving)

175 calories

8g fat

21g carbohydrates

7g protein

Chickpeas have the ideal balance of protein and also high quality carbohydrate to maintain blood glucose levels steady, which also can help keep inflammation at bay. This crispy, savory snack remains lower in sodium using spices which provide antioxidant packed taste, therefore less salt is necessary. Additionally, the pinch is really gratifying!

Ingredients

1, 15-ounce may chickpeas

3 tsp olive oil

1 tsp lime juice

2 tsp tsp powder

1/2 tsp garlic powder

1/2 tsp paprika

1/4 tsp salt

Preparation

1. Pre-heat oven to 400 f.

2. Rinse and drain chickpeas and blot with a paper towel to remove moisture. Do not bypass this step or your own chickpeas will not get overly eloquent.

3. Toss chickpeas using 1.5 tsp of olive oil and set onto a foil-lined baking sheet.

4. Bake in 400 degrees for 25 seconds. Remove from oven and let it cool completely on the baking sheet.

5. Switch oven down to 350 f.

6. Stir collectively remaining 1.5 tsp oil, lime juice, carrot, garlic, paprika, and salt until it forms a paste.

7. Toss mix with heated chickpeas and use your hands to guarantee all of chickpeas are all coated.

8. Spread chickpeas evenly on the exact same foil-lined baking sheet and bake in 350 f for about 15 minutes, checking them every 5 minutes to be certain they are burning.

9. Allow chickpeas to cool before eating. If the chickpeas are completed, they ought to feel lighter and also be quite crunchy but not burnt. Store them in an airtight container at room temperature for as much as two days. But they are best eaten straight away.

Fixing variations and substitutions

Ditch the final item with lime zest to include much more lime taste, and a bit little longer of fiber.

Try eucalyptus oil rather than olive oil to switch the taste. The change will not significantly influence the nutrition profile as most oils have approximately the exact same number of fat and calories each level. Sesame oil and olive oil equally comprise healthy mono- and - poly-unsaturated carbohydrates, which can be useful for decreasing inflammation.

If you are short on time, then substitute chili powder and salt for the spices. The salt count will be greater in this instance.

Craving a cheesy bite? Replace cumin using 1 tbsp grated parmesan cheese, that adds 2 g of protein, also calcium, for just 20 calories .

Cooking and serving tips

The greater you blot the chickpeas, the crispier that they get. Also, be certain to cool the chickpeas entirely between roasting cycles to make certain they get emptied instead of mushy.

Split into individual portions and shop in zip-top snack luggage to get a convenient anti inflammatory bite on-the-go or on the job.

Stovetop apple cinnamon popcorn

Complete time: 10 minutes

Prep time: 5 minutes

Cook time: 5 minutes

Servings: 2 servings (2 cups per day)

Nutrition highlights (per serving)

154 calories

9g fat

18g carbohydrates

2g protein

Popcorn is a fast and tasty snack that is easy to create when the craving strikes. The issue with some popcorn, such as microwave popcorn, is the fact that it's frequently loaded with salt and butter, each of which may mean difficulty for your cardiovascular health. But, popcorn can be a entire grain, meaning it's packed with fiber and is excellent for helping to reduce your blood pressure. The secret is popping up and flavoring your popcorn using heart-healthy ingredients.

This apple cinnamon popcorn is popped to the stove together with heart-healthy petroleum . It's actually quite simple to create if you have never attempted popping popcorn on the stove. It's pitched with cinnamon and citrus processors to get a yummy, fall-inspired deal with.

Ingredients

1 tbsp canola or avocado

2 tbsp unpopped popcorn kernels

3/4 tsp cinnamon

1/2 cup apple chips

Preparation

1. Heating petroleum in a small saucepan over moderate heat. Insert a couple of popcorn kernels into the pan.

2. After they pop, add remaining popcorn into the pan. Cover the lid and shake till you notice the popping up slow. Watch attentively as popcorn may burn off fast.

3. Eliminate from heat and add cinnamon and berries. Toss to coat. Pour into bowls for serving.

Fixing variations and substitutions

Consider adding ground ginger, nutmeg, or cloves

for much more spice.

Try out banana chips, dried lemon dried or dried mango pieces instead of the apple chips to get a tropical popcorn mixture. When picking, make certain that there's no extra sugar.

If you want a savory combination, consider incorporating beet or carrot fries and peppermint spices like chili powder, paprika, pepper, or garlic powder.

Cooking and serving tips

This popcorn is excellent for snacking during your next film night or for packaging together with you to munch on when you're on the move. Experiment with various spices and dried fruit to seek out your favourite flavor blend.

Watch popcorn attentively while still popping. It may burn quickly! It's normal to have a couple of unpopped kernels at the base.

Be attentive when discovering popped popcorn. There'll be hot steam .

Dessert

Indulge and revel in sweet treats with no dairy.

Vegan grilled sweet and spicy pineapple

Complete time: 15 minutes

Prep time: 10 minutes

Cook time: 5 minutes

Servings: 6

Nutrition highlights (per serving)

123 calories

4g fat

24g carbohydrates

1g protein

Fruit for dessert? Boooring! But maybe not with this particular recipe for broiled sweet and hot pineapple. Sprinkled with a little bit of spiced sugar and drizzled with rich almond milk, so it has got the ideal blend of tastes and textures.

Ingredients

1 pineapple, peeled, cored, and chopped

2 tsp raw sugar

1/8 tsp cayenne

1/8 tsp salt

4 tbsp almond milk

3 lime wedges

1 tbsp toasted coconut flakes, optional, for garnish

Preparation

1. Oil grates of a barbecue. Place to medium-high warmth. When hot, put lemon slices on the grill and cook 2-3 minutes each side until lightly charred. Eliminate lemon into a plate.

2. In a little bowl, blend together sugar, cayenne, and salt. Sprinkle over the lemon. Drizzle with almond milk. Spritz with lemon juice. When utilizing, sprinkle with coconut aromas. Serve hot or room temperature.

Fixing variations and substitutions

Grilled fruit really is a sin! Popping fruit onto a hot

grill gently caramelizes the face area, brings out it is natural sweetness, also gives it a touch of sour flavor. If your fruit is not very mature, it is a wonderful way to bring out more sweetness and flavor. Try this process with peas, cantaloupe, peaches, mangos, or peanuts.

Is the blood glucose sensitive to your fruit? For a few with diabetes, then the fiber is sufficient to avoid a spike in blood glucose in the naturally occurring sugar levels. But other people, particularly those with more complex diabetes, might be more sensitive. If that is the situation, like a smaller quantity over yogurt. The fat and protein from the yogurt can keep blood sugar steady. Or you can swap your treasured non-caloric sweetener or leave the sugar out entirely.

If you are concerned about the spice, then use a smaller quantity of saltwater or switch to spicy crushed red pepper aromas. Or you can use cinnamon, that is not hot but adds a different layer of special taste. As a bonus, as it also helps reduce blood glucose.

Cooking and serving tips

To make sure that your fruit does not burn off, make sure that your grill is fine and clean. Leftover pieces of charred food onto the grates may add a sour, unpleasant taste to the dish.

This recipe is ideal for serving in picnics or outdoor fun. If had to conserve grill the fruit beforehand and refrigerate until ready to work with. Then top with all the hot sugar, coconut milk, and lime before serving.

To make this dish decadent, best with dark chocolate chips, sliced toasted cashews, and shredded coconut.

Gluten-free cinnamon lemon coconut bliss balls recipe

Complete time: 8 minutes

Prep time: 8 minutes

Cook time: 0 minute

Servings: 20

Nutrition highlights (per serving)

97 calories

8g fat

6g carbohydrates

3g protein

Word of caution: those cinnamon lemon citrus bliss balls are so somewhat addictive. But that is okay because every individual has only under 100 calories and just 3 g of sugar so you're able to use your best judgment about when to gratify.

Wish to understand the secret to maintaining the sugar low? The odd but yummy traces of cinnamon and lemon zest. If you like lemon and cinnamon and you have never attempted this combo ahead, you will be addicted!

Besides being low in sugar, they are also a fantastic source of heart-healthy mono and polyunsaturated fats. Additionally, they are super easy to create? The toughest part would be zesting the lemon, however you may still be noshing in under 10 seconds flat--ideal once you're craving just a little something sweet!

Ingredients

2 cups nice almond milk

1/4 cup pure maple syrup

2 tbsp coconut oil

2 tsp lemon zest, or to flavor

1 tsp ground cinnamon, or to taste

1/4 tsp sea salt or table salt

1/4 cup shredded unsweetened coconut

Preparation

1. Blend almond milk, maple syrup, vanilla oil, lemon zest, cinnamon, and salt in a microwave . Process until mixture is well blended and slightly tacky.

2. Line a massive plate small baking sheet with plastic wrap and then divide dough into 20 pieces. Roll each slice into a ball.

3. Place shredded coconut onto a little plate and roll each ball from the coconut, and then come back into plate or baking sheet. May function immediately or

store covered in refrigerator until ready to consume.

Fixing variations and substitutions

You can substitute the coconut oil for any impartial tasting vegetable oil liquid coconut oil. Don't hesitate to add extra lemon zest and coconut oil if needed. Start with recommended quantities, then add more as required.

Cooking and serving tips

You may make a large batch of them and keep them at a well-sealed container in the freezer. Love them suspended, or thaw them a bit from the fridge prior to serving. These bliss balls are fantastic for an afternoon treat with a cup of java.

Mocha dusted almonds: a satisfying, chocolatey snack

Complete time: 10 minutes

Prep time: 5 minutes

Cook time: 5 minutes

Servings: 6 (1 oz each)

Nutrition highlights (per serving)

148 calories

13g fat

6g carbohydrates

5g protein

Satisfying snacks must be approximately 150 to 250 calories and include a mixture of protein, fiber, also healthful fats. All these mocha dusted almonds supply three to your greatest tasty snack that can stick together till your meal. The coffee taste enhances the cherry to provide you a deep chocolate taste in little serving.

Research has shown that the flavonols found in anti aging are capable of reducing blood pressure if consumed as part of an overall healthier diet. Cocoa also contains potassium, calcium magnesium, magnesium and aluminum, all which play a part in keeping a wholesome blood pressure. Cocoa also includes a substantial quantity of phosphorus and iron. Unsweetened cocoa powder is particularly beneficial since it doesn't have sugar or fat.

Next time you're craving something crunchy or sweet, whip up a pile of these to delight in weekly. Only 1 recipe makes enough for one to part out to 6 portions for easy snacking every moment!

Ingredients

1 cup raw almonds (unsalted)

1/2 tsp extra virgin olive oil

1 tbsp unsweetened cocoa powder

1 tsp instant coffee granules

1 tsp powdered sugar

Preparation

1. In a tiny skillet, toast almonds over low heat, stirring every few seconds, until they are aromatic, about 3 minutes. Add olive oil and stir to coat. Remove from heat.

2. Combination cocoa powder, coffee, and sugar at

a high powered blender or food processor until the java granules are integrated into a powder.

3. Pour almonds and ginger mixture to a medium bowl and toss to coat evenly. Shake off excess. Distribute over parchment or waxed paper to cool.

4. Shop almonds in a airtight container at room temperature.

Fixing variations and substitutions

If you want a diabetes-friendly edition, replace sugar with 1/4 into 1/2 tsp stevia.

Use this recipe with any nuts that you would like, just make certain they're raw, not roasted and salted, to maintain the salt material on the reduced side.

Cooking and serving tips

I love to utilize dutch processed cocoa or dark chocolate raspberry powder to get a rich chocolate flavor, however any unsweetened cocoa powder works nicely.

Portion ready cakes out beforehand to stash on your luggage or car to get a healthful snack on the move! Doing so will also keep you from consuming more than the recommended serving size.

Cooking and meal planning

Changing into a vegetarian diet gets easier after you become familiar with the wide selection of foods which are available to you with this diet. Focusing on the meals that you may consume aids divert your focus from the foods that you can not eat.

Occurs with vegan alternatives

If you are a dairy enthusiast, there are lots of vegetarian choices that you can utilize. Utilize nut milk cereal and in java rather than cow's milk or cream. You may even milk-alternatives in recipes which call for milk milk, but you might choose to use unflavored types. Some state that rice has a consistency nearest to cow's milk.

If you like cheese, start looking for artisan manufacturers which make alternative products from components such as ginseng, shiro, miso paste, garlic, and other seasonings. You could also locate cheese produced from tapioca. Remember, however, that curry cheese does not always act like milk cheese . Some detect a difference in how it melts. A lot of individuals also use supplement, a deactivated yeast using a pleasant, nutty flavor which makes it particularly helpful in producing pasta dishes or cheese sauces.

If you like a hearty breakfast, then scramble tofu just like you'd typically scramble eggs. Top it with dinner to get a spicy kick. Additionally, there are vegan egg replacements for baking and cooking.

Many companies create sausage from vegetables such as eggplant and fennel together with significant grains. Use whole grain bread to make pancakes and other breakfast meals subsequently utilize pure maple syrup rather than honey as a sweetener.

Plan ahead

Cooking foods beforehand may help you adapt to your vegetarian diet--particularly if you're utilized to eating foods. Having ingredients prepared to go will make it a lot easier for you to gather a snack or meal quickly when you are hungry.

- Cook and bake beans daily weekly. Keep them refrigerated so you are able to catch a few to throw on on top of noodles to get a fast protein boost.

- Soak oats immediately therefore they are all set to cook fast in the daytime.

- Chop vegetables and fruits beforehand and maintain them single-serving containers that they are all set to catch when you want a bite.

CHAPTER EIGHT

THE VEGAN GUIDE

FOODS TO EAT ON A VEGAN DIET

VEGETABLES
Artichoke

Arugula

Asparagus

Beet

Broccoli

Brussel Sprouts

Cabbage

Carrots

Cauliflower

Celery

Collard Greens

Cucumber

Endives

Fennel

Garlic

Kale

Leek

Lettuce

Mushrooms

Mustard Greens

Okra

Onions

Parsnip

Peppers

Potatoes

Radish

Rhubarb

Spinach

Squashes

Tomato

Zucchini

FRUITS

Apples

Avocado

Bananas

Blackberries

Blueberries

Dates

Grapefruit

Grapes

Kiwi

Lemon

Lime

Mango

Melon

Orange

Peach

Pear

Pineapple

Pomegranate

Strawberries

Raspberries

Water Melon

SEEDS

Chia

Flax

Hemp

Pumpkin

Quinoa

Sesame

Sunflower

BEANS & LEGUMES

Bean Sprouts

Black Beans

Black-Eyed Peas

Butter Beans

Chickpeas

Green Beans

Kidney Beans

Lentils

Mung Beans

Navy Beans

Peanuts

Pinto Beans

Soy Beans

GRAINS

Barley

Bran

Buckwheat

Bulgur

Couscous

Kamut

Millet

Orzo

Spelt

Corn

Rice

Rye

Oats

Teff

Wheat

HERBS & SPICES

Basil

Cilantro/Coriander

Dill

Fennel

Oregano

Paprika

Parsley

Rosemary

Sage

Thyme

NUTS

Almonds

Brazil Nuts

Cashews

Chestnuts

Hazelnuts

Pecans

Pine Nuts

Macadamias

Pistachios

Walnuts

TOP VEGAN SWAPS

Milk   —>   Almond Milk

Cream —>   Coconut Cream

Butter —>   Olive Oil

Cheese —>   Nutritional Yeast

Eggs   —>   Flax Egg

Meat   —>   Tempeh

Honey —>Agave Syrup

Ice Cream —>Frozen Bananas

TOP VEGAN PROTEIN SOURCES

Tempeh

Soy Beans

Lentils

Black Beans

Kidney Beans

Veggies Burgers

Chickpeas

Tofu

Quinoa

Peanut Butter

Almonds

Pumpkin Seeds

SPOTLIGHT ON SOY

Soy is a popular and sometimes controversial ingredient; it is derived from the soy bean legume. A complete protein and rich in calcium, iron, zinc, fiber and potassium. Soy can replace dairy and/or meat in the diet although it may be considered a health food, not all soy products are created equal.

Soy products, both fermented and unfermented, range in their degree of processing, from soy flour and soy protein to more traditional foods like miso, soy milk and tofu. Highly processed items to avoid include soy cheese, soy yoghurt and imitation meats. Focus on traditional forms to maintain the soy's nutrient density.

TOP SOY PRODUCTS

Miso

A thick pasta made from fermented soy beans, rice or barley malt.

Soy Milk

Finely ground up soy beans, soaked and strained to produce a milky liquid.

Tofu

Soy bean curds.

Tempeh

Whole soy beans fermented into a cake or patty.

Edamame

Whole, green soy bean.

CHAPTER NINE

28 DAYS DIET PLAN FOR FIREFIGHTERS

DAY ONE

Breakfast

Green Protein Smoothie

INGREDIENTS

- 1/2 Frozen Banana

- 1 Cup of Spinach

- 1 Avocado

- 1 Serving of Vanilla Protein Powder

- 1 Cup of Almond Milk

- 1 Tbsp of Chia Seeds

DIRECTIONS

1. Start by pouring the almond milk into the blender to avoid the ingredients sticking at the bottom of the blender.

2. Next add in the banana, avocado, spinach, chia seeds and the protein powder.

3. Turn the blender on, starting at a low speed and increase as needed.

4. Once the liquid looks even, pour into a cup and enjoy immediately to conserve as many nutrients as possible.

NUTRITIONAL VALUE (per serving)

Fat: 20 g

Carbs: 28 g

Protein: 42 g

Total Calories: 430 Calories

Lunch

Chickpea Wrap

INGREDIENTS

- 1 Brown Rice Tortilla Wraps

- 1 Cup of Chickpeas

- 1/2 Avocado

- 1 Stalks of Celery

- 1/4 Cup of Red Onions

- 2 Tbsp of Vegan Mayo

- Pinch of Sea Salt and Ground Pepper

DIRECTIONS

1. Wash and drain the chickpeas. Put the chickpeas in a big bowl and mash them with a fork.

2. Chop the celery and red onion into small pieces and add it to the chickpeas.

3. Toss in the remaining of the ingredients.

4. Divide the mixture up into two separate wraps.

NUTRITIONAL VALUE

Fat: 36 g

Carbs: 45 g

Protein: 15 g

Total Calories: 631 Calories

Dinner

Vegan Power Bowl

INGREDIENTS (2 Servings)

- 2 Cups Kale

- 1 Roasted Sweet Potato

- 1 Avocado

- 1 Red Bell Pepper

- 1 Can of Black Bean

- 1 tsp of Olive Oil

- Dressing:

- 2 Tbsp of Tahini

- 2 Tbsp of Lemon Juice

DIRECTIONS

1. Pre-heat the oven at 350F/175C. Place the cube sized sweet potatoes on a baking tray with parchment paper and bake for 30 minutes.

2. While the sweet potatoes are baking, clean and chop up the kale. Once the kale is ready mix it in with the olive oil and massage it into the kale.

3. Chop the red pepper and avocado. Prepare the dressing by mixing the tahini and the fresh lemon juice together.

4. Once the sweet potatoes are done, place the massaged kale at the bottom of a dish and add all of the other ingredients on top of it and finish it off with the dressing.

NUTRITIONAL VALUE (per serving)

Fat: 33 g

Carbs: 67 g

Protein: 21 g

Total Calories: 599 Calories

Snacks

Hummus & Cucumber Sticks

INGREDIENTS (4 servings)

- 1 Can of Chickpeas

- 1/4 Cup of Tahini

- 2 Tbsp of Extra Virgin Olive Oil

- 2 Tbsp of Lemon Juice

- 1 Clove of Garlic

- 1 tsp of Cumin

- 1/2 tsp of Sea Salt

- 1 Cup of Cucumber Sticks

DIRECTIONS

1. Start by preparing the chickpeas. If you are preparing dry chickpeas follow the instructions on the packaging or if you are using canned make sure to drain the chickpeas and rinse them well.

2. Once the chickpeas are ready, place all of the ingredients in a food processor and process until it forms a smooth and creamy texture.

3. Store the hummus into an air tight container or portion it out immediately into 4 servings.

NUTRITIONAL VALUE (per serving)

Fat: 16 g

Carbs: 22 g

Protein: 8 g

Total Calories: 251 Calories

DAY TWO

Breakfast

Superfood Oatmeal

INGREDIENTS

- 1/2 Cup of Gluten Free

- Oatmeal

- 1 Cup of Almond Milk

- 1/4 Cup of Almonds

- 1/2 Cup of Berries

- 1 tsp of Ground Cinnamon

DIRECTIONS

1. In a pot place the oats, cinnamon and the almond milk and turn the heat on high until it starts boiling.

2. Once it is boiling turn the heat down to low and stir until all of the almond milk is absorbed.

3. Once the oatmeal is ready transfer it into a bowl and add the nuts and fresh berries.

4. Optional: Add honey or extra toppings.

NUTRITIONAL VALUE

Fat: 21 g

Carbs: 40 g

Protein: 12 g

Total Calories: 401 Calories

Lunch

Vegan Power Bowl (leftovers)

INGREDIENTS (2 Servings)

- 2 Cups Kale

- 1 Roasted Sweet Potato

- 1 Avocado

- 1 Red Bell Pepper

- 1 Can of Black Bean

- 1 tsp of Olive Oil

- Dressing:

- 2 Tbsp of Tahini

- 2 Tbsp of Lemon Juice

DIRECTIONS

1. Pre-heat the oven at 350F/175C. Place the cube sized sweet potatoes on a baking tray with parchment paper and bake for 30 minutes.

2. While the sweet potatoes are baking, clean and chop up the kale. Once the kale is ready mix it in with the olive oil and massage it into the kale.

3. Chop the red pepper and avocado. Prepare the dressing by mixing the tahini and the fresh lemon juice together.

4. Once the sweet potatoes are done, place the massaged kale at the bottom of a dish and add all of the other ingredients on top of it and finish it off with the dressing.

NUTRITIONAL VALUE (per serving)

Fat: 33 g

Carbs: 67 g

Protein: 21 g

Total Calories: 599 Calories

Dinner

Balsamic Arugula Salad

INGREDIENTS (2 Servings)

- 4 Cups of Arugula

- 2 Tomatoes

- 1 Cup of Chopped Cucumber

- 1 Cup of Chickpeas

- 2 Tbsp of Balsamic Vinegar

- 1/4 Cup of Extra Virgin Olive Oil

- Pinch of Sea Salt and Pepper

DIRECTIONS

1. Pre-heat the oven to 200C/400F.

2. Drain and wash the chickpeas and then pat them dry with a paper towel. Spread the chickpeas out on

a baking sheet with parchment paper and drizzle the 2 Tbsp of olive oil on top. Bake the chickpeas for 30 minutes, moving them around every 10 minutes.

3. While the chickpeas are baking prepare the salad ingredients. Make the dressing by combining the balsamic vinegar, olive oil, sea salt and pepper.

4. You can add a sweetener of choice here as well if desired.

5. Once the chickpeas are done toss them into the prepared salad for a much healthier crouton alternative.

NUTRITIONAL VALUE (per serving)

Fat: 29 g

Carbs: 28 g

Protein: 6 g

Total Calories: 391 Calories

Snacks

Cacao Coconut Balls

INGREDIENTS (Makes 10 Balls)

- 1 Cup of Almonds

- 1/2 Cup of Shredded Coconut

- 8 Medjool Dates

- 2 Tbsp of Raw Cacao Powder

DIRECTIONS

1. Remove the pit from the dates. Combine all the ingredients in a food processor and mix until it forms a doughy mixture.

2. Form 10 balls with the mixture and then store them into the fridge to preserve freshness.

NUTRITIONAL VALUE (2 balls)

Fat: 18 g

Carbs: 36 g

Protein: 6 g

Total Calories: 324 Calories

DAY THREE

Breakfast

Green Protein Smoothie

INGREDIENTS

- 1/2 Frozen Banana

- 1 Cup of Spinach

- 1 Avocado

- 1 Serving of Vanilla Protein Powder

- 1 Cup of Almond Milk

- 1 Tbsp of Chia Seeds

DIRECTIONS

1. Start by pouring the almond milk into the blender to avoid the ingredients sticking at the bottom of the blender.

2. Next add in the banana, avocado, spinach, chia seeds and the protein powder.

3. Turn the blender on, starting at a low speed and increase as needed.

4. Once the liquid looks even, pour into a cup and enjoy immediately to conserve as many nutrients as

possible.

NUTRITIONAL VALUE (per serving)

Fat: 20 g

Carbs: 28 g

Protein: 42 g

Total Calories: 430 Calories

Lunch

Balsamic Arugula Salad (leftovers)

INGREDIENTS (2 Servings)

- 4 Cups of Arugula

- 2 Tomatoes

- 1 Cup of Chopped Cucumber

- 1 Cup of Chickpeas

- 2 Tbsp of Balsamic Vinegar

- 1/4 Cup of Extra Virgin Olive Oil

- Pinch of Sea Salt and Pepper

DIRECTIONS

1. Pre-heat the oven to 200C/400F.

2. Drain and wash the chickpeas and then pat them dry with a paper towel. Spread the chickpeas out on a baking sheet with parchment paper and drizzle the 2 Tbsp of olive oil on top. Bake the chickpeas for 30 minutes, moving them around every 10 minutes.

3. While the chickpeas are baking prepare the salad ingredients. Make the dressing by combining the balsamic vinegar, olive oil, sea salt and pepper.

4. You can add a sweetener of choice here as well if desired.

5. Once the chickpeas are done toss them into the prepared salad for a much healthier crouton alternative.

NUTRITIONAL VALUE (per serving)

Fat: 29 g

Carbs: 28 g

Protein: 6 g

Total Calories: 391 Calories

Dinner

Portobello Fajita Bowl

INGREDIENTS (2 Servings)

- 2 Portobello Mushroom

- 1 Red Bell Pepper

- 1/4 Cup of Onions

- 2 Cloves of Garlic

- 1/2 Cup of Brown Rice

- 1/2 Cup of Guacamole

- Fajita Seasoning:

- 2 Tbsp of Paprika

- 1 Tbsp of Garlic Powder

- 1 Tbsp of Onion Powder

- 1 tsp of Cayenne Powder

DIRECTIONS

1. Place a pan on medium heat and add the coconut oil.

2. Once the oil has melted add the onions and garlic and sauté for 1 minute.

3. Next add the red pepper and portobello mushroom cut into long thin slices.

4. Add the fajita seasoning and cook for another 5-7 minutes.

5. Meanwhile prepare the guacamole.

6. Once everything is ready combine the Portobello mixture, brown rice and guacamole in a big bowl.

NUTRITIONAL VALUE (per serving)

Fat: 19 g

Carbs: 46 g

Protein: 8 g

Total Calories: 390 Calories

Snacks

Hummus & Cucumber Sticks

INGREDIENTS (4 servings)

- 1 Can of Chickpeas

- 1/4 Cup of Tahini

- 2 Tbsp of Extra Virgin Olive Oil

- 2 Tbsp of Lemon Juice

- 1 Clove of Garlic

- 1 tsp of Cumin

- 1/2 tsp of Sea Salt

- 1 Cup of Cucumber Sticks

DIRECTIONS

1. Start by preparing the chickpeas. If you are preparing dry chickpeas follow the instructions on the packaging or if you are using canned make sure to drain the chickpeas and rinse them well.

2. Once the chickpeas are ready, place all of the ingredients in a food processor and process until it forms a smooth and creamy texture.

3. Store the hummus into an air tight container or portion it out immediately into 4 servings.

NUTRITIONAL VALUE (per serving)

Fat: 16 g

Carbs: 22 g

Protein: 8 g

Total Calories: 251 Calories

DAY FOUR

Breakfast

Superfood Oatmeal

INGREDIENTS

- 1/2 Cup of Gluten Free

- Oatmeal

- 1 Cup of Almond Milk

- 1/4 Cup of Almonds

- 1/2 Cup of Berries

- 1 tsp of Ground Cinnamon

DIRECTIONS

1. In a pot place the oats, cinnamon and the almond milk and turn the heat on high until it starts boiling.

2. Once it is boiling turn the heat down to low and stir until all of the almond milk is absorbed.

3. Once the oatmeal is ready transfer it into a bowl and add the nuts and fresh berries.

4. Optional: Add honey or extra toppings.

NUTRITIONAL VALUE

Fat: 21 g

Carbs: 40 g

Protein: 12 g

Total Calories: 401 Calories

Lunch

Portobello Fajita Bowl (leftovers)

Portobello Fajita Bowl

INGREDIENTS (2 Servings)

- 2 Portobello Mushroom

- 1 Red Bell Pepper

- 1/4 Cup of Onions

- 2 Cloves of Garlic

- 1/2 Cup of Brown Rice

- 1/2 Cup of Guacamole

- Fajita Seasoning:

- 2 Tbsp of Paprika

- 1 Tbsp of Garlic Powder

- 1 Tbsp of Onion Powder

- 1 tsp of Cayenne Powder

DIRECTIONS

1. Place a pan on medium heat and add the coconut oil.

2. Once the oil has melted add the onions and garlic and sauté for 1 minute.

3. Next add the red pepper and portobello mushroom cut into long thin slices.

4. Add the fajita seasoning and cook for another 5-7 minutes.

5. Meanwhile prepare the guacamole.

6. Once everything is ready combine the Portobello mixture, brown rice and guacamole in a big bowl.

NUTRITIONAL VALUE (per serving)

Fat: 19 g

Carbs: 46 g

Protein: 8 g

Total Calories: 390 Calories

Dinner

Tofu Pad Thai

INGREDIENTS (2 Servings)

- 8 oz of Tofu

- 4 oz of Brown Rice Noodles

- 1 Cup of Bean Sprouts

- 1/2 Cup of Green Onions

- 1 Cloves of Garlic

- 1/4 Cup of Coconut Aminos

- 2 Tbsp of Almond Butter

- 1 Tbsp of Coconut Oil

DIRECTIONS

1. Place a pan on medium heat and add the coconut oil.

2. Finely chop the garlic and onions and place it in the pan with the cubed tofu. While the tofu is sautéing, fill up a pot with water and bring to a boil.

3. Once the water is boiling add the brown rice noodles.

4. When the tofu is starting to brown add in the bean sprouts.

5. Mix together the coconut aminos and the almond butter to form a thick sauce and toss it in the pan and lower the heat.

6. Cook for another 5 minutes.

7. Once the tofu and the noodles are ready, combine them in a plate.

8. Add the fresh green onions on top.

NUTRITIONAL VALUE (per serving)

Fat: 26 g

Carbs: 58 g

Protein: 24 g

Total Calories: 485 Calories

Snacks

Cacao Coconut Balls

INGREDIENTS (Makes 10 Balls)

- 1 Cup of Almonds

- 1/2 Cup of Shredded Coconut

- 8 Medjool Dates

- 2 Tbsp of Raw Cacao Powder

DIRECTIONS

1. Remove the pit from the dates. Combine all the ingredients in a food processor and mix until it forms a doughy mixture.

2. Form 10 balls with the mixture and then store them into the fridge to preserve freshness.

NUTRITIONAL VALUE (2 balls)

Fat: 18 g

Carbs: 36 g

Protein: 6 g

Total Calories: 324 Calories

DAY FIVE

Breakfast

Green Protein Smoothie

INGREDIENTS

- 1/2 Frozen Banana

- 1 Cup of Spinach

- 1 Avocado

- 1 Serving of Vanilla Protein Powder

- 1 Cup of Almond Milk

- 1 Tbsp of Chia Seeds

DIRECTIONS

1. Start by pouring the almond milk into the blender to avoid the ingredients sticking at the bottom of the

blender.

2. Next add in the banana, avocado, spinach, chia seeds and the protein powder.

3. Turn the blender on, starting at a low speed and increase as needed.

4. Once the liquid looks even, pour into a cup and enjoy immediately to conserve as many nutrients as possible.

NUTRITIONAL VALUE (per serving)

Fat: 20 g

Carbs: 28 g

Protein: 42 g

Total Calories: 430 Calories

Lunch

Tofu Pad Thai (leftovers)

INGREDIENTS (2 Servings)

- 8 oz of Tofu

- 4 oz of Brown Rice Noodles

- 1 Cup of Bean Sprouts

- 1/2 Cup of Green Onions

- 1 Cloves of Garlic

- 1/4 Cup of Coconut Aminos

- 2 Tbsp of Almond Butter

- 1 Tbsp of Coconut Oil

DIRECTIONS

1. Place a pan on medium heat and add the coconut oil.

2. Finely chop the garlic and onions and place it in the pan with the cubed tofu. While the tofu is sautéing, fill up a pot with water and bring to a boil.

3. Once the water is boiling add the brown rice noodles.

4. When the tofu is starting to brown add in the bean sprouts.

5. Mix together the coconut aminos and the almond butter to form a thick sauce and toss it in the pan

and lower the heat.

6. Cook for another 5 minutes.

7. Once the tofu and the noodles are ready, combine them in a plate.

8. Add the fresh green onions on top.

NUTRITIONAL VALUE (per serving)

Fat: 26 g

Carbs: 58 g

Protein: 24 g

Total Calories: 485 Calories

Dinner

Eat Out Using the Vegan Guide Guidelines

Snacks

Hummus & Cucumber Sticks

INGREDIENTS (4 servings)

- 1 Can of Chickpeas

- 1/4 Cup of Tahini

- 2 Tbsp of Extra Virgin Olive Oil

- 2 Tbsp of Lemon Juice

- 1 Clove of Garlic

- 1 tsp of Cumin

- 1/2 tsp of Sea Salt

- 1 Cup of Cucumber Sticks

DIRECTIONS

1. Start by preparing the chickpeas. If you are preparing dry chickpeas follow the instructions on the packaging or if you are using canned make sure to drain the chickpeas and rinse them well.

2. Once the chickpeas are ready, place all of the ingredients in a food processor and process until it forms a smooth and creamy texture.

3. Store the hummus into an air tight container or portion it out immediately into 4 servings.

NUTRITIONAL VALUE (per serving)

Fat: 16 g

Carbs: 22 g

Protein: 8 g

Total Calories: 251 Calories

DAY SIX

Breakfast

Superfood Oatmeal

INGREDIENTS

- 1/2 Cup of Gluten Free

- Oatmeal

- 1 Cup of Almond Milk

- 1/4 Cup of Almonds

- 1/2 Cup of Berries

- 1 tsp of Ground Cinnamon

DIRECTIONS

1. In a pot place the oats, cinnamon and the almond milk and turn the heat on high until it starts boiling.

2. Once it is boiling turn the heat down to low and

stir until all of the almond milk is absorbed.

3. Once the oatmeal is ready transfer it into a bowl and add the nuts and fresh berries.

4. Optional: Add honey or extra toppings.

NUTRITIONAL VALUE

Fat: 21 g

Carbs: 40 g

Protein: 12 g

Total Calories: 401 Calories

Lunch

Rainbow Salad

INGREDIENTS

- 1 Cup of Spinach

- 1/2 Zucchini (Preferably Spiralized)

- 1/2 Cup of Shredded Carrots

- 1/2 Cup of Shredded Red Cabbage

- Dressing:

- 1/2 Avocado

- 2 Tbsp of Extra Virgin Olive Oil

- Juice of 1/2 Lime

DIRECTIONS

1. Prepare all of the vegetables as listed above. I highly recommend creating different textures with your vegetables to add variety.

2. Place the mixed greens at the bottom of the bowl then add all of the vegetables on top. Combine the avocado, extra virgin olive oil and the lime juice with salt and pepper to create a creamy dressing.

3. Serve with the dressing drizzled on top.

NUTRITIONAL VALUE

Fat: 42 g

Carbs: 23 g

Protein: 3 g

Total Calories: 457 Calories

Dinner

Sweet Potato Chickpea Curry

INGREDIENTS

- (2 Servings)

- 1.5 Cup (1 Small) of Sweet Potato

- 1 Can of Chickpeas

- 1 Cup of Coconut Milk

- 1/4 Cup of Onion

- 1 Can of Chopped Tomato

- 1 Tbsp of Olive Oil

- 1 Tbsp of Ground Turmeric

- 1 Tbsp of Ground Cumin

- 1 Tbsp of Ground Ginger

- 1 tsp of Sea Salt

DIRECTIONS

1. In a large pot heat the olive oil and the onions and the spices. Cook until the onions become translucent.

2. Next add in the rest of the ingredients, making sure that the sweet potatoes are completely covered with the liquid.

3. Bring the curry to a boil and then turn down to a simmer for about 40 minutes or until the sweet potatoes are completely done.

NUTRITIONAL VALUE (per serving)

Fat: 26 g

Carbs: 56 g

Protein: 13 g

Total Calories: 518 Calories

Snacks

Cacao Coconut Balls

INGREDIENTS (Makes 10 Balls)

- 1 Cup of Almonds

- 1/2 Cup of Shredded Coconut

- 8 Medjool Dates

- 2 Tbsp of Raw Cacao Powder

DIRECTIONS

1. Remove the pit from the dates. Combine all the ingredients in a food processor and mix until it forms a doughy mixture.

2. Form 10 balls with the mixture and then store them into the fridge to preserve freshness.

NUTRITIONAL VALUE (2 balls)

Fat: 18 g

Carbs: 36 g

Protein: 6 g

Total Calories: 324 Calories

DAY SEVEN

Breakfast

Banana Pancakes

INGREDIENTS

- 1 Cup of Gluten Free Oatmeal

- 1/4 Cup of Almond Milk

- 1 Banana

- 1 Tbsp of Coconut Oil

- 2 tsp of Baking Powder

- 1/2 tsp of Cinnamon

DIRECTIONS

1. In a bowl combine all of the ingredients except for the coconut oil. Use a hand blender or a fork to mix everything together. Aim for a consistency similar to pancake batter.

2. Place a pan on medium heat and melt the coconut oil. Slowly add the batter in the pan forming 5 inch diameter pancakes. Place the cover on and cook for a couple minutes on each side.

3. Repeat until you have cooked the whole batch. Be creative with your toppings, add any of your favourite clean foods. These may include but are not limited to berries, almond butter, coconut flakes and chopped nuts.

NUTRITIONAL VALUE

Fat: 24 g

Carbs: 30 g

Protein: 14 g

Total Calories: 378 Calories

Lunch

Sweet Potato Chickpea Curry (leftovers)

INGREDIENTS

- (2 Servings)

- 1.5 Cup (1 Small) of Sweet Potato

- 1 Can of Chickpeas

- 1 Cup of Coconut Milk

- 1/4 Cup of Onion

- 1 Can of Chopped Tomato

- 1 Tbsp of Olive Oil

- 1 Tbsp of Ground Turmeric

- 1 Tbsp of Ground Cumin

- 1 Tbsp of Ground Ginger

- 1 tsp of Sea Salt

DIRECTIONS

1. In a large pot heat the olive oil and the onions and the spices. Cook until the onions become translucent.

2. Next add in the rest of the ingredients, making sure that the sweet potatoes are completely covered with the liquid.

3. Bring the curry to a boil and then turn down to a simmer for about 40 minutes or until the sweet potatoes are completely done.

NUTRITIONAL VALUE (per serving)

Fat: 26 g

Carbs: 56 g

Protein: 13 g

Total Calories: 518 Calories

Dinner

Mexican Stuffed Peppers

INGREDIENTS (2 Servings)

- 2 Red Bell Peppers

- 1/4 Cup of Quinoa

- 1/2 Cup of Black Beans

- 1/2 Cup of Salsa

- 1/4 Cup of Fresh Chopped

- Cilantro

- 1 tsp of Paprika

- 1 tsp of Chili Powder

- Pinch of Sea Salt & Pepper

DIRECTIONS

1. Pre-heat the oven to 350F/175C and bake the peppers for 10 minutes on a baking tray.

2. Meanwhile cook the quinoa according to the directions on the packaging.

3. Mix all of the ingredients into a bowl then take the red pepper out of the oven and stuff them with

the mixture.

4. Place the stuffed peppers back on the baking sheet and bake for another 10 minutes.

NUTRITIONAL VALUE (per serving)

Fat: 2 g

Carbs: 44 g

Protein: 12 g

Total Calories: 238 Calories

Snacks

Hummus & Cucumber Sticks

INGREDIENTS (4 servings)

- 1 Can of Chickpeas

- 1/4 Cup of Tahini

- 2 Tbsp of Extra Virgin Olive Oil

- 2 Tbsp of Lemon Juice

- 1 Clove of Garlic

- 1 tsp of Cumin

- 1/2 tsp of Sea Salt

- 1 Cup of Cucumber Sticks

DIRECTIONS

1. Start by preparing the chickpeas. If you are preparing dry chickpeas follow the instructions on the packaging or if you are using canned make sure to drain the chickpeas and rinse them well.

2. Once the chickpeas are ready, place all of the ingredients in a food processor and process until it forms a smooth and creamy texture.

3. Store the hummus into an air tight container or portion it out immediately into 4 servings.

NUTRITIONAL VALUE (per serving)

Fat: 16 g

Carbs: 22 g

Protein: 8 g

Total Calories: 251 Calories

WEEK TWO

DAY ONE

Breakfast

Raspberry Coconut Smoothie

INGREDIENTS

- 1 Cup of Blueberries

- 1 Banana

- 1 Cup of Coconut Milk

- 1 Serving of Vanilla Protein Powder

- Handful of Ice

DIRECTIONS

1. Start by pouring the coconut milk into the blender to avoid the ingredients sticking at the bottom of the blender.

2. Next, throw in the blueberries, banana, collagen powder and the ice. Turn the blender on, starting at a low speed and increase as needed.

3. Once the liquid looks even, pour into a cup and enjoy immediately to conserve as many nutrients as

possible.

NUTRITIONAL VALUE

Fat: 18 g

Carbs: 53 g

Protein: 20 g

Total Calories: 436 Calories

Lunch

Mexican Stuffed Peppers (leftovers)

INGREDIENTS (2 Servings)

- 2 Red Bell Peppers

- 1/4 Cup of Quinoa

- 1/2 Cup of Black Beans

- 1/2 Cup of Salsa

- 1/4 Cup of Fresh Chopped

- Cilantro

- 1 tsp of Paprika

- 1 tsp of Chili Powder

- Pinch of Sea Salt & Pepper

DIRECTIONS

1. Pre-heat the oven to 350F/175C and bake the peppers for 10 minutes on a baking tray.

2. Meanwhile cook the quinoa according to the directions on the packaging.

3. Mix all of the ingredients into a bowl then take the red pepper out of the oven and stuff them with the mixture.

4. Place the stuffed peppers back on the baking sheet and bake for another 10 minutes.

NUTRITIONAL VALUE (per serving)

Fat: 2 g

Carbs: 44 g

Protein: 12 g

Total Calories: 238 Calories

Dinner

Creamy Avocado Pasta

INGREDIENTS (2 Servings)

- 4 oz of Brown Rice Linguini

- 1 Avocado

- 1/2 Cup of Fresh Basil

- 2 Tbsp of Extra Virgin Olive Oil

- 2 Cloves of Garlic

- 1 Tbsp of Lemon Juice

- Pinch of Sea Salt and Pepper

DIRECTIONS

1. Start by preparing the pasta according to the directions on the packaging.

2. While the pasta is cooking start preparing the avocado cream sauce by combining all of the ingredients in a food processor.

3. Process until the consistency is nice and smooth.

4. Add the avocado cream sauce with the noodles once they are ready.

5. Feel free to add to favourite vegetarian protein

source to this dish if you prefer a meal with higher protein.

NUTRITIONAL VALUE (per serving)

Fat: 27 g

Carbs: 47 g

Protein: 7 g

Total Calories: 446 Calories

Snacks

Seed Crackers & Guacamole

INGREDIENTS (Makes 4 Servings)

- 1/4 Cup of Chia Seeds

- 1/4 Cups of Sesame Seeds

- 1/4 Cups of Sunflower Seeds

- 1/2 Tbsp of Herb Mix Seasoning

- 1/2 tsp of Sea Salt

- 1 Cup of Water

Guacamole:

- 1/2 Mashed Avocado

- Juice of Half a Lime

- Pinch of Sea Salt

DIRECTIONS

1. Preheat the oven to 175C.

2. Combine all the seeds together with water and seasonings. Let the mixture sit for 5 minutes.

3. Line a baking sheet with parchment paper and spread the seed mixture evenly until flat.

4. Bake for 30 minutes then remove from the oven, cut them into squares, flip them and bake for another

15 minutes.

5. Meanwhile combine the guacamole ingredients in a bowl and mash until you have your desired consistency.

DAY TWO

Breakfast

Chocolate Overnight Oats

INGREDIENTS

- 1/2 Cup of Gluten Free Oatmeal

- 1 Cup of Almond Milk

- 1 Serving of Chocolate Protein Powder

- 1 Tbsp of Chia Seeds

- 1 Tbsp of Raw Cacao Powder

- 1 Tbsp of Maple Syrup

Optional: Raw Cacao Nibs

DIRECTIONS

1. Combine all the ingredients into a mason jar or a sealed container, give it a good stir and place in the fridge overnight.

2. In the morning, add raw cacao nibs on top for an extra crunch if desired.

3. Enjoy cold or heated up.

NUTRITIONAL VALUE

Fat: 18 g

Carbs: 60 g

Protein: 46 g

Total Calories: 550 Calories

Lunch

Creamy Avocado Pasta (leftovers)

INGREDIENTS (2 Servings)

- 4 oz of Brown Rice Linguini
- 1 Avocado
- 1/2 Cup of Fresh Basil
- 2 Tbsp of Extra Virgin Olive Oil
- 2 Cloves of Garlic
- 1 Tbsp of Lemon Juice
- Pinch of Sea Salt and Pepper

DIRECTIONS

1. Start by preparing the pasta according to the directions on the packaging.

2. While the pasta is cooking start preparing the avocado cream sauce by combining all of the ingredients in a food processor.

3. Process until the consistency is nice and smooth.

4. Add the avocado cream sauce with the noodles once they are ready.

5. Feel free to add to favourite vegetarian protein source to this dish if you prefer a meal with higher protein.

NUTRITIONAL VALUE (per serving)

Fat: 27 g

Carbs: 47 g

Protein: 7 g

Total Calories: 446 Calories

Dinner

Falafel Salad

INGREDIENTS (2 Servings)

- 1 Can of Chickpeas

- 1/4 Cup of Red Onion

- 1/2 Cup of Fresh Parsley

- 1 Cloves of Garlic

- 1/2 tsp of Cumin

- Pinch of Sea Salt & Pepper

- 2 Cup of Fresh Greens

- 2 Tbsp of Tahini

- 1 tsp of Lemon Juice

DIRECTIONS

1. Pre-heat the oven to 400F.

2. Combine the chickpeas, red onions, garlic, cumin, parsley and cilantro in a food processor. Process for a few seconds, leaving the mixture a little bit chunky.

3. Form 8 small patties with the mixture and then refrigerate for an hour to let them set.

4. Bake for 45 minutes, flipping them half way.

5. While the falafel are baking prepare the salad and

the dressing by combining the tahini and lemon juice.

NUTRITIONAL VALUE (4 Falafel)

Fat: 3 g

Carbs: 29 g

Protein: 9 g

Total Calories: 171 Calories

Snacks

Carrots & Almond Butter

INGREDIENTS

- 2 Carrots

- 1 Tbsp of Almond Butter

DIRECTIONS

1. Slice the carrots into sticks and use the almond butter as a dip.

NUTRITIONAL VALUE

Fat: 19 g

Carbs: 13 g

Protein: 5 g

Total Calories: 229 Calories

DAY THREE

Breakfast

Raspberry Coconut Smoothie

INGREDIENTS

- 1 Cup of Blueberries

- 1 Banana

- 1 Cup of Coconut Milk

- 1 Serving of Vanilla Protein Powder

- Handful of Ice

DIRECTIONS

1. Start by pouring the coconut milk into the blender to avoid the ingredients sticking at the bottom of the blender.

2. Next, throw in the blueberries, banana, collagen powder and the ice. Turn the blender on, starting at

a low speed and increase as needed.

3. Once the liquid looks even, pour into a cup and enjoy immediately to conserve as many nutrients as possible.

NUTRITIONAL VALUE

Fat: 18 g

Carbs: 53 g

Protein: 20 g

Total Calories: 436 Calories

Lunch

Falafel Salad (leftovers)

INGREDIENTS (2 Servings)

- 1 Can of Chickpeas

- 1/4 Cup of Red Onion

- 1/2 Cup of Fresh Parsley

- 1 Cloves of Garlic

- 1/2 tsp of Cumin

- Pinch of Sea Salt & Pepper

- 2 Cup of Fresh Greens

- 2 Tbsp of Tahini

- 1 tsp of Lemon Juice

DIRECTIONS

1. Pre-heat the oven to 400F.

2. Combine the chickpeas, red onions, garlic, cumin, parsley and cilantro in a food processor. Process for a few seconds, leaving the mixture a little bit chunky.

3. Form 8 small patties with the mixture and then refrigerate for an hour to let them set.

4. Bake for 45 minutes, flipping them half way.

5. While the falafel are baking prepare the salad and the dressing by combining the tahini and lemon juice.

NUTRITIONAL VALUE (4 Falafel)

Fat: 3 g

Carbs: 29 g

Protein: 9 g

Total Calories: 171 Calories

Dinner

Tofu Almond Butter Stir Fry

INGREDIENTS (2 Servings)

- 8 oz of Tofu

- 2 Cups of Broccoli

- 1 Red Bell Pepper

- 4 Mushrooms

- 1/4 Cup of Red Onion

- 2 Tbsp of Coconut Oil

- Almond Butter Sauce:

- 1/4 Cup of Coconut Aminos

- 2 Tbsp of Almond Butter

DIRECTIONS

1. Chop all the vegetables in bite size pieces.

2. In a large pan place the coconut oil and the tofu cubed on medium heat and cook for a few minutes.

3. Once the tofu has begun to brown a little bit add all of the chopped vegetables and the sauce and cook for another 5-10 minutes (depending on how you like your vegetables).

4. Turn the heat off, take the cover off and let the sauce thicken up for a few minutes before serving.

NUTRITIONAL VALUE (per serving)

Fat: 43 g

Carbs: 49 g

Protein: 25 g

Total Calories: 563 Calories

Snacks

Seed Crackers & Guacamole

INGREDIENTS (Makes 4 Servings)

- 1/4 Cup of Chia Seeds

- 1/4 Cups of Sesame Seeds

- 1/4 Cups of Sunflower Seeds

- 1/2 Tbsp of Herb Mix Seasoning

- 1/2 tsp of Sea Salt

- 1 Cup of Water

Guacamole:

- 1/2 Mashed Avocado

- Juice of Half a Lime

- Pinch of Sea Salt

DIRECTIONS

1. Preheat the oven to 175C.

2. Combine all the seeds together with water and seasonings. Let the mixture sit for 5 minutes.

3. Line a baking sheet with parchment paper and spread the seed mixture evenly until flat.

4. Bake for 30 minutes then remove from the oven, cut them into squares, flip them and bake for another

15 minutes.

5. Meanwhile combine the guacamole ingredients in a bowl and mash until you have your desired consistency.

DAY FOUR

Breakfast

Chocolate Overnight Oats

INGREDIENTS

- 1/2 Cup of Gluten Free Oatmeal

- 1 Cup of Almond Milk

- 1 Serving of Chocolate Protein Powder

- 1 Tbsp of Chia Seeds

- 1 Tbsp of Raw Cacao Powder

- 1 Tbsp of Maple Syrup

Optional: Raw Cacao Nibs

DIRECTIONS

1. Combine all the ingredients into a mason jar or a sealed container, give it a good stir and place in the fridge overnight.

2. In the morning, add raw cacao nibs on top for an extra crunch if desired.

3. Enjoy cold or heated up.

NUTRITIONAL VALUE

Fat: 18 g

Carbs: 60 g

Protein: 46 g

Total Calories: 550 Calories

Lunch

Tofu Almond Butter Stir Fry (leftovers)

INGREDIENTS (2 Servings)

- 8 oz of Tofu

- 2 Cups of Broccoli

- 1 Red Bell Pepper

- 4 Mushrooms

- 1/4 Cup of Red Onion

- 2 Tbsp of Coconut Oil

- Almond Butter Sauce:

- 1/4 Cup of Coconut Aminos

- 2 Tbsp of Almond Butter

DIRECTIONS

1. Chop all the vegetables in bite size pieces.

2. In a large pan place the coconut oil and the tofu cubed on medium heat and cook for a few minutes.

3. Once the tofu has begun to brown a little bit add all of the chopped vegetables and the sauce and cook for another 5-10 minutes (depending on how you like your vegetables).

4. Turn the heat off, take the cover off and let the sauce thicken up for a few minutes before serving.

NUTRITIONAL VALUE (per serving)

Fat: 43 g

Carbs: 49 g

Protein: 25 g

Total Calories: 563 Calories

Dinner

Black Bean Burgers

INGREDIENTS (2 Servings)

- 1 Can of Black Beans

- 1/4 Cup of Gluten Free Oatmeal

- 1/4 Cup of Chopped Onion

- 2 Cloves of Garlic

- 1/4 Cup of Fresh Parsley

- 1 tsp of Chilli

- 1/2 tsp of Cayenne Powder

- 1/2 tsp of Sea Salt

- 1/2 tsp of Pepper

DIRECTIONS

1. Drain and rinse the black beans and pat dry with paper towel.

2. Place all of the ingredients in a food processor and the mixture becomes sticky.

3. Form 4 patties and cook on the stove top on medium heat with coconut oil.

4. Fry the patty for about 3-5 minutes each side and then you can add any of your favourite toppings to the burger patties.

NUTRITIONAL VALUE (2 Patties)

Fat: 2 g

Carbs: 46 g

Protein: 16 g

Total Calories: 262 Calories

Snacks

Carrots & Almond Butter

INGREDIENTS

- 2 Carrots

- 1 Tbsp of Almond Butter

DIRECTIONS

1. Slice the carrots into sticks and use the almond butter as a dip.

NUTRITIONAL VALUE

Fat: 19 g

Carbs: 13 g

Protein: 5 g

Total Calories: 229 Calories

DAY FIVE

Breakfast

Raspberry Coconut Smoothie

INGREDIENTS

- 1 Cup of Blueberries

- 1 Banana

- 1 Cup of Coconut Milk

- 1 Serving of Vanilla Protein Powder

- Handful of Ice

DIRECTIONS

1. Start by pouring the coconut milk into the blender to avoid the ingredients sticking at the bottom of the

blender.

2. Next, throw in the blueberries, banana, collagen powder and the ice. Turn the blender on, starting at a low speed and increase as needed.

3. Once the liquid looks even, pour into a cup and enjoy immediately to conserve as many nutrients as possible.

NUTRITIONAL VALUE

Fat: 18 g

Carbs: 53 g

Protein: 20 g

Total Calories: 436 Calories

Lunch

Black Bean Burgers (leftovers)

INGREDIENTS (2 Servings)

- 1 Can of Black Beans

- 1/4 Cup of Gluten Free Oatmeal

- 1/4 Cup of Chopped Onion

- 2 Cloves of Garlic

- 1/4 Cup of Fresh Parsley

- 1 tsp of Chilli

- 1/2 tsp of Cayenne Powder

- 1/2 tsp of Sea Salt

- 1/2 tsp of Pepper

DIRECTIONS

1. Drain and rinse the black beans and pat dry with paper towel.

2. Place all of the ingredients in a food processor and the mixture becomes sticky.

3. Form 4 patties and cook on the stove top on medium heat with coconut oil.

4. Fry the patty for about 3-5 minutes each side and then you can add any of your favourite toppings to the burger patties.

NUTRITIONAL VALUE (2 Patties)

Fat: 2 g

Carbs: 46 g

Protein: 16 g

Total Calories: 262 Calories

Dinner

Eat Out Using the Vegan Guide Guidelines

Snacks

Seed Crackers & Guacamole

INGREDIENTS (Makes 4 Servings)

- 1/4 Cup of Chia Seeds

- 1/4 Cups of Sesame Seeds

- 1/4 Cups of Sunflower Seeds

- 1/2 Tbsp of Herb Mix Seasoning

- 1/2 tsp of Sea Salt

- 1 Cup of Water

Guacamole:

- 1/2 Mashed Avocado

- Juice of Half a Lime

- Pinch of Sea Salt

DIRECTIONS

1. Preheat the oven to 175C.

2. Combine all the seeds together with water and seasonings. Let the mixture sit for 5 minutes.

3. Line a baking sheet with parchment paper and spread the seed mixture evenly until flat.

4. Bake for 30 minutes then remove from the oven, cut them into squares, flip them and bake for another

15 minutes.

5. Meanwhile combine the guacamole ingredients in a bowl and mash until you have your desired consistency.

DAY SIX

Breakfast

Chocolate Overnight Oats

INGREDIENTS

- 1/2 Cup of Gluten Free Oatmeal

- 1 Cup of Almond Milk

- 1 Serving of Chocolate Protein Powder

- 1 Tbsp of Chia Seeds

- 1 Tbsp of Raw Cacao Powder

- 1 Tbsp of Maple Syrup

Optional: Raw Cacao Nibs

DIRECTIONS

1. Combine all the ingredients into a mason jar or a sealed container, give it a good stir and place in the fridge overnight.

2. In the morning, add raw cacao nibs on top for an extra crunch if desired.

3. Enjoy cold or heated up.

NUTRITIONAL VALUE

Fat: 18 g

Carbs: 60 g

Protein: 46 g

Total Calories: 550 Calories

Lunch

Crunchy Kale Salad

INGREDIENTS

- 2 Cups of Kale

- 1 Carrot

- 1/2 Avocado

- 1/2 Cup of Chickpeas

- Dressing:

- 1 Tbsp of Tahini

- 1 Tbsp of Lemon Juice

DIRECTIONS

1. Preheat the oven to 350F/175C.

2. Drain and rinse the chickpeas. Dry them with a paper towel and spread them evenly on a baking tray. Bake for 45 minutes.

3. Meanwhile prepare the vegetables by rinsing and chopping up the kale, peeling and shredding the carrots and cutting the avocado into small cubes. Set the vegetables aside.

4. Combine all the dressing ingredients into a bowl and whisk together until it forms a smooth consistency.

5. Place all of the vegetables to a bowl with the baked chickpeas and then drizzle the dressing on top.

NUTRITIONAL VALUE

Fat: 22 g

Carbs: 40 g

Protein: 16 g

Total Calories: 431 Calories

Dinner

Zoodles & Lentil Meatballs

INGREDIENTS (2 Servings)

- 2 Zucchinis

- 1 Cup of Cooked Lentils

- 1/4 Cup of Quinoa

- 1/2 Cup of Almond Flour

- 1/4 Cup of Chopped Onion

- 2 Garlic Cloves

- 2 Tbsp of Italian Seasoning

- 400 ml of Marinara Sauce

DIRECTIONS

1. Start by preparing the lentils and quinoa according to directions on the package.

2. Once the lentils and quinoa are ready add everything except for the marinara sauce and zucchini in the food processor.

3. Process until it is completely smooth. Roll out 10 small "meatballs" with the lentil mixture.

4. Heat olive oil in a large pan and cook the meatballs for 5 minutes.

5. Next add the marinara sauce to the pan, mix in

with the meatballs and cook for another 5 minutes.

6. Serve over spiralized zucchini. If you do not have a spiralizer you can create linguini noodles out of zucchini with a regular peeler.

NUTRITIONAL VALUE (per serving)

Fat: 18 g

Carbs: 55 g

Protein: 20 g

Total Calories: 441 Calories

Snacks

Carrots & Almond Butter

INGREDIENTS

- 2 Carrots

- 1 Tbsp of Almond Butter

DIRECTIONS

1. Slice the carrots into sticks and use the almond butter as a dip.

NUTRITIONAL VALUE

Fat: 19 g

Carbs: 13 g

Protein: 5 g

Total Calories: 229 Calories

DAY SEVEN

Breakfast

Banana Pancakes

INGREDIENTS

- 1 Cup of Gluten Free Oatmeal

- 1/4 Cup of Almond Milk

- 1 Banana

- 1 Tbsp of Coconut Oil

- 2 tsp of Baking Powder

- 1/2 tsp of Cinnamon

DIRECTIONS

1. In a bowl combine all of the ingredients except for the coconut oil. Use a hand blender or a fork to

mix everything together. Aim for a consistency similar to pancake batter.

2. Place a pan on medium heat and melt the coconut oil. Slowly add the batter in the pan forming 5 inch diameter pancakes. Place the cover on and cook for a couple minutes on each side.

3. Repeat until you have cooked the whole batch. Be creative with your toppings, add any of your favourite clean foods. These may include but are not limited to berries, almond butter, coconut flakes and chopped nuts.

NUTRITIONAL VALUE

Fat: 24 g

Carbs: 30 g

Protein: 14 g

Total Calories: 378 Calories

Lunch

Zoodles & Lentil Meatballs (leftovers)

Zoodles & Lentil Meatballs

INGREDIENTS (2 Servings)

- 2 Zucchinis

- 1 Cup of Cooked Lentils

- 1/4 Cup of Quinoa

- 1/2 Cup of Almond Flour

- 1/4 Cup of Chopped Onion

- 2 Garlic Cloves

- 2 Tbsp of Italian Seasoning

- 400 ml of Marinara Sauce

DIRECTIONS

1. Start by preparing the lentils and quinoa according to directions on the package.

2. Once the lentils and quinoa are ready add everything except for the marinara sauce and zucchini in the food processor.

3. Process until it is completely smooth. Roll out 10 small "meatballs" with the lentil mixture.

4. Heat olive oil in a large pan and cook the

meatballs for 5 minutes.

5. Next add the marinara sauce to the pan, mix in with the meatballs and cook for another 5 minutes.

6. Serve over spiralized zucchini. If you do not have a spiralizer you can create linguini noodles out of zucchini with a regular peeler.

NUTRITIONAL VALUE (per serving)

Fat: 18 g

Carbs: 55 g

Protein: 20 g

Total Calories: 441 Calories

Dinner

Quinoa Tabouleh

INGREDIENTS

- 1/4 Cup of Quinoa

- 1/2 Cup of Fresh Parsley

- 2 Tomatoes

- 2 Tbsp of Pine Nuts

- 1 Tbsp of Tahini

- 1 Tbsp of Olive Oil

- Juice of 1/2 Lemon

DIRECTIONS

1. Start by preparing the quinoa according to the directions on the packaging.

2. While the quinoa is cooking start chopping the parsley and the tomatoes.

3. Once the quinoa is done let it cool down for a little bit and then add all of the remaining ingredients.

4. Mix well and serve cold.

NUTRITIONAL VALUE

Fat: 29 g

Carbs: 36 g

Protein: 10 g

Total Calories: 423 Calories

Snacks

Seed Crackers & Guacamole

INGREDIENTS (Makes 4 Servings)

- 1/4 Cup of Chia Seeds

- 1/4 Cups of Sesame Seeds

- 1/4 Cups of Sunflower Seeds

- 1/2 Tbsp of Herb Mix Seasoning

- 1/2 tsp of Sea Salt

- 1 Cup of Water

Guacamole:

- 1/2 Mashed Avocado

- Juice of Half a Lime

- Pinch of Sea Salt

DIRECTIONS

1. Preheat the oven to 175C.

2. Combine all the seeds together with water and seasonings. Let the mixture sit for 5 minutes.

3. Line a baking sheet with parchment paper and

spread the seed mixture evenly until flat.

4. Bake for 30 minutes then remove from the oven, cut them into squares, flip them and bake for another

15 minutes.

5. Meanwhile combine the guacamole ingredients in a bowl and mash until you have your desired consistency.

WEEK THREE

DAY ONE

Breakfast

Chocolate Banana Smoothie

INGREDIENTS

- 1 Frozen Banana

- 1/2 Avocado

- 1 Cup of Almond Milk

- 2 Tbsp of Raw Cacao Powder

- 1 Serving Chocolate Protein Powder

DIRECTIONS

1. Start by pouring the almond milk into the blender to avoid the ingredients sticking at the bottom of the blender.

2. Next, throw in the banana, avocado, cacao powder and the protein powder. Turn the blender on, starting at a low speed and increase as needed.

3. Once the liquid is even pour into a cup and enjoy immediately to conserve as many nutrients as possible.

NUTRITIONAL VALUE

Fat: 10 g

Carbs: 54 g

Protein: 41 g

Total Calories: 448 Calories

Lunch

Chicken Wrap

INGREDIENTS

- 1 Brown Rice Tortilla Wraps

- 1 Cup of Chickpeas

- 1/2 Avocado

- 1 Stalks of Celery

- 1/4 Cup of Red Onions

- 2 Tbsp of Vegan Mayo

- Pinch of Sea Salt and Ground Pepper

DIRECTIONS

1. Wash and drain the chickpeas. Put the chickpeas in a big bowl and mash them with a fork.

2. Chop the celery and red onion into small pieces and add it to the chickpeas.

3. Toss in the remaining of the ingredients.

4. Divide the mixture up into two separate wraps.

NUTRITIONAL VALUE

Fat: 36 g

Carbs: 45 g

Protein: 15 g

Total Calories: 631 Calories

Dinner

Vegan Power Bowl

INGREDIENTS (2 Servings)

- 2 Cups Kale

- 1 Roasted Sweet Potato

- 1 Avocado

- 1 Red Bell Pepper

- 1 Can of Black Bean

- 1 tsp of Olive Oil

- Dressing:

- 2 Tbsp of Tahini

- 2 Tbsp of Lemon Juice

DIRECTIONS

1. Pre-heat the oven at 350F/175C. Place the cube sized sweet potatoes on a baking tray with

parchment paper and bake for 30 minutes.

2. While the sweet potatoes are baking, clean and chop up the kale. Once the kale is ready mix it in with the olive oil and massage it into the kale.

3. Chop the red pepper and avocado. Prepare the dressing by mixing the tahini and the fresh lemon juice together.

4. Once the sweet potatoes are done, place the massaged kale at the bottom of a dish and add all of the other ingredients on top of it and finish it off with the dressing.

NUTRITIONAL VALUE (per serving)

Fat: 33 g

Carbs: 67 g

Protein: 21 g

Total Calories: 599 Calories

Snacks

Coconut Chia Pudding

INGREDIENTS (4 Servings)

- 1 Can of Coconut Milk

- 1/4 Cup of Chia Seeds

- 1 Tbsp of Maple Syrup

- 1 tsp of Vanilla Extract

- 1 Cup of Berries

DIRECTIONS

1. Combine all of the ingredients in a bowl except the berries. Stir well and then transfer the mixture to a sealed container.

2. Let the chia seed pudding sit in the refrigerator for

3 hours or overnight.

3. Once it is ready you can separate it into 4 servings and add a handful of berries on top.

NUTRITIONAL VALUE (per serving)

Fat: 25 g

Carbs: 14 g

Protein: 5 g

Total Calories: 299 Calories

DAY TWO

Breakfast

Tofu Scrambles

INGREDIENTS

- 4oz of Tofu

- 1/2 Cup of Red Bell Pepper

- 1 Cup of Spinach

- 1/4 Cup of Red Onion

- 1 Tbsp of Coconut Aminos

- 1 tsp of Coconut Oil

- 1 tsp of Turmeric

- 1/2 tsp of Sea Salt

- Pinch of Black Pepper

DIRECTIONS

1. Place a pan on medium heat and add the onions
and peppers with the coconut oil.

2. Once the vegetables become translucent add the tofu to the pan and roughly break it down with a spatula.

3. Next add the coconut aminos, turmeric, salt and pepper and cook for another 5 minutes.

4. Add the spinach in the last 2 minutes to avoid wilting too much.

5. Enjoy!

NUTRITIONAL VALUE

Fat: 14 g

Carbs: 12 g

Protein: 15 g

Total Calories: 173 Calories

Lunch

Vegan Power Bowl (Laftovers)

INGREDIENTS (2 Servings)

- 2 Cups Kale

- 1 Roasted Sweet Potato

- 1 Avocado

- 1 Red Bell Pepper

- 1 Can of Black Bean

- 1 tsp of Olive Oil

- Dressing:

- 2 Tbsp of Tahini

- 2 Tbsp of Lemon Juice

DIRECTIONS

1. Pre-heat the oven at 350F/175C. Place the cube sized sweet potatoes on a baking tray with parchment paper and bake for 30 minutes.

2. While the sweet potatoes are baking, clean and chop up the kale. Once the kale is ready mix it in with the olive oil and massage it into the kale.

3. Chop the red pepper and avocado. Prepare the dressing by mixing the tahini and the fresh lemon juice together.

4. Once the sweet potatoes are done, place the

massaged kale at the bottom of a dish and add all of the other ingredients on top of it and finish it off with the dressing.

NUTRITIONAL VALUE (per serving)

Fat: 33 g

Carbs: 67 g

Protein: 21 g

Total Calories: 599 Calories

Dinner

Balsamic Arugula Salad

INGREDIENTS (2 Servings)

- 4 Cups of Arugula

- 2 Tomatoes

- 1 Cup of Chopped Cucumber

- 1 Cup of Chickpeas

- 2 Tbsp of Balsamic Vinegar

- 1/4 Cup of Extra Virgin Olive Oil

- Pinch of Sea Salt and Pepper

DIRECTIONS

1. Pre-heat the oven to 200C/400F.

2. Drain and wash the chickpeas and then pat them dry with a paper towel. Spread the chickpeas out on a baking sheet with parchment paper and drizzle the 2 Tbsp of olive oil on top. Bake the chickpeas for 30 minutes, moving them around every 10 minutes.

3. While the chickpeas are baking prepare the salad ingredients. Make the dressing by combining the balsamic vinegar, olive oil, sea salt and pepper.

4. You can add a sweetener of choice here as well if desired.

5. Once the chickpeas are done toss them into the prepared salad for a much healthier crouton alternative.

NUTRITIONAL VALUE (per serving)

Fat: 29 g

Carbs: 28 g

Protein: 6 g

Total Calories: 391 Calories

Snacks

Coconut Chia Pudding

INGREDIENTS (4 Servings)

- 1 Can of Coconut Milk

- 1/4 Cup of Chia Seeds

- 1 Tbsp of Maple Syrup

- 1 tsp of Vanilla Extract

- 1 Cup of Berries

DIRECTIONS

1. Combine all of the ingredients in a bowl except the berries. Stir well and then transfer the mixture to a sealed container.

2. Let the chia seed pudding sit in the refrigerator for

3 hours or overnight.

3. Once it is ready you can separate it into 4

servings and add a handful of berries on top.

NUTRITIONAL VALUE (per serving)

Fat: 25 g

Carbs: 14 g

Protein: 5 g

Total Calories: 299 Calories

DAY THREE

Breakfast

Chocolate Banana Smoothie

INGREDIENTS

- 1 Frozen Banana

- 1/2 Avocado

- 1 Cup of Almond Milk

- 2 Tbsp of Raw Cacao Powder

- 1 Serving Chocolate Protein Powder

DIRECTIONS

1. Start by pouring the almond milk into the blender

to avoid the ingredients sticking at the bottom of the blender.

2. Next, throw in the banana, avocado, cacao powder and the protein powder. Turn the blender on, starting at a low speed and increase as needed.

3. Once the liquid is even pour into a cup and enjoy immediately to conserve as many nutrients as possible.

NUTRITIONAL VALUE

Fat: 10 g

Carbs: 54 g

Protein: 41 g

Total Calories: 448 Calories

Lunch

Balsamic Arugula Salad (Leftovers)

INGREDIENTS (2 Servings)

- 4 Cups of Arugula

- 2 Tomatoes

- 1 Cup of Chopped Cucumber

- 1 Cup of Chickpeas

- 2 Tbsp of Balsamic Vinegar

- 1/4 Cup of Extra Virgin Olive Oil

- Pinch of Sea Salt and Pepper

DIRECTIONS

1. Pre-heat the oven to 200C/400F.

2. Drain and wash the chickpeas and then pat them dry with a paper towel. Spread the chickpeas out on a baking sheet with parchment paper and drizzle the 2 Tbsp of olive oil on top. Bake the chickpeas for 30 minutes, moving them around every 10 minutes.

3. While the chickpeas are baking prepare the salad ingredients. Make the dressing by combining the balsamic vinegar, olive oil, sea salt and pepper.

4. You can add a sweetener of choice here as well if desired.

5. Once the chickpeas are done toss them into the prepared salad for a much healthier crouton

alternative.

NUTRITIONAL VALUE (per serving)

Fat: 29 g

Carbs: 28 g

Protein: 6 g

Total Calories: 391 Calories

Dinner

Portobello Fajita Bowl

INGREDIENTS (2 Servings)

- 2 Portobello Mushroom

- 1 Red Bell Pepper

- 1/4 Cup of Onions

- 2 Cloves of Garlic

- 1/2 Cup of Brown Rice

- 1/2 Cup of Guacamole

- Fajita Seasoning:

- 2 Tbsp of Paprika

- 1 Tbsp of Garlic Powder

- 1 Tbsp of Onion Powder

- 1 tsp of Cayenne Powder

DIRECTIONS

1. Place a pan on medium heat and add the coconut oil.

2. Once the oil has melted add the onions and garlic and sauté for 1 minute.

3. Next add the red pepper and portobello mushroom cut into long thin slices.

4. Add the fajita seasoning and cook for another 5-7 minutes.

5. Meanwhile prepare the guacamole.

6. Once everything is ready combine the Portobello mixture, brown rice and guacamole in a big bowl.

NUTRITIONAL VALUE (per serving)

Fat: 19 g

Carbs: 46 g

Protein: 8 g

Total Calories: 390 Calories

Snacks

Coconut Chia Pudding

INGREDIENTS (4 Servings)

- 1 Can of Coconut Milk

- 1/4 Cup of Chia Seeds

- 1 Tbsp of Maple Syrup

- 1 tsp of Vanilla Extract

- 1 Cup of Berries

DIRECTIONS

1. Combine all of the ingredients in a bowl except the berries. Stir well and then transfer the mixture to a sealed container.

2. Let the chia seed pudding sit in the refrigerator for

3 hours or overnight.

3. Once it is ready you can separate it into 4

servings and add a handful of berries on top.

NUTRITIONAL VALUE (per serving)

Fat: 25 g

Carbs: 14 g

Protein: 5 g

Total Calories: 299 Calories

DAY FOUR

Breakfast

Tofu Scrambles

INGREDIENTS

- 4oz of Tofu

- 1/2 Cup of Red Bell Pepper

- 1 Cup of Spinach

- 1/4 Cup of Red Onion

- 1 Tbsp of Coconut Aminos

- 1 tsp of Coconut Oil

- 1 tsp of Turmeric

- 1/2 tsp of Sea Salt

- Pinch of Black Pepper

DIRECTIONS

1. Place a pan on medium heat and add the onions and peppers with the coconut oil.

2. Once the vegetables become translucent add the tofu to the pan and roughly break it down with a spatula.

3. Next add the coconut aminos, turmeric, salt and pepper and cook for another 5 minutes.

4. Add the spinach in the last 2 minutes to avoid wilting too much.

5. Enjoy!

NUTRITIONAL VALUE

Fat: 14 g

Carbs: 12 g

Protein: 15 g

Total Calories: 173 Calories

Lunch

Portobello Fajita Bowl (Leftovers)

INGREDIENTS (2 Servings)

- 2 Portobello Mushroom

- 1 Red Bell Pepper

- 1/4 Cup of Onions

- 2 Cloves of Garlic

- 1/2 Cup of Brown Rice

- 1/2 Cup of Guacamole

- Fajita Seasoning:

- 2 Tbsp of Paprika

- 1 Tbsp of Garlic Powder

- 1 Tbsp of Onion Powder

- 1 tsp of Cayenne Powder

DIRECTIONS

1. Place a pan on medium heat and add the coconut oil.

2. Once the oil has melted add the onions and garlic and sauté for 1 minute.

3. Next add the red pepper and portobello mushroom cut into long thin slices.

4. Add the fajita seasoning and cook for another 5-7 minutes.

5. Meanwhile prepare the guacamole.

6. Once everything is ready combine the Portobello mixture, brown rice and guacamole in a big bowl.

NUTRITIONAL VALUE (per serving)

Fat: 19 g

Carbs: 46 g

Protein: 8 g

Total Calories: 390 Calories

Dinner

Tofu Pad Thai

INGREDIENTS (2 Servings)

- 8 oz of Tofu

- 4 oz of Brown Rice Noodles

- 1 Cup of Bean Sprouts

- 1/2 Cup of Green Onions

- 1 Cloves of Garlic

- 1/4 Cup of Coconut Aminos

- 2 Tbsp of Almond Butter

- 1 Tbsp of Coconut Oil

DIRECTIONS

1. Place a pan on medium heat and add the coconut oil.

2. Finely chop the garlic and onions and place it in the pan with the cubed tofu. While the tofu is sautéing, fill up a pot with water and bring to a boil.

3. Once the water is boiling add the brown rice noodles.

4. When the tofu is starting to brown add in the bean sprouts.

5. Mix together the coconut aminos and the almond

butter to form a thick sauce and toss it in the pan and lower the heat.

6. Cook for another 5 minutes.

7. Once the tofu and the noodles are ready, combine them in a plate.

8. Add the fresh green onions on top.

NUTRITIONAL VALUE (per serving)

Fat: 26 g

Carbs: 58 g

Protein: 24 g

Total Calories: 485 Calories

Snacks

Apple Pie Bites

INGREDIENTS (10 balls)

- 8 Medjool Dates

- 1 Cup of Dried Apples

- 1 Cup of Walnuts

- 1 tsp of Cinnamon

DIRECTIONS

1. Remove the pit from the dates. Combine all the ingredients in a food processor and mix until it forms a doughy mixture.

2. Form 10 balls with the mixture.

NUTRITIONAL VALUE (2 Balls)

Fat: 16 g

Carbs: 44 g

Protein: 5 g

Total Calories: 314 Calories

DAY FIVE

Breakfast

Chocolate Banana Smoothie

Chocolate Banana Smoothie

INGREDIENTS

- 1 Frozen Banana

- 1/2 Avocado

- 1 Cup of Almond Milk

- 2 Tbsp of Raw Cacao Powder

- 1 Serving Chocolate Protein Powder

DIRECTIONS

1. Start by pouring the almond milk into the blender to avoid the ingredients sticking at the bottom of the blender.

2. Next, throw in the banana, avocado, cacao powder and the protein powder. Turn the blender on, starting at a low speed and increase as needed.

3. Once the liquid is even pour into a cup and enjoy immediately to conserve as many nutrients as possible.

NUTRITIONAL VALUE

Fat: 10 g

Carbs: 54 g

Protein: 41 g

Total Calories: 448 Calories

Lunch

Tofu Pad Thai (leftovers)

INGREDIENTS (2 Servings)

- 8 oz of Tofu

- 4 oz of Brown Rice Noodles

- 1 Cup of Bean Sprouts

- 1/2 Cup of Green Onions

- 1 Cloves of Garlic

- 1/4 Cup of Coconut Aminos

- 2 Tbsp of Almond Butter

- 1 Tbsp of Coconut Oil

DIRECTIONS

1. Place a pan on medium heat and add the coconut oil.

2. Finely chop the garlic and onions and place it in the pan with the cubed tofu. While the tofu is

sautéing, fill up a pot with water and bring to a boil.

3. Once the water is boiling add the brown rice noodles.

4. When the tofu is starting to brown add in the bean sprouts.

5. Mix together the coconut aminos and the almond butter to form a thick sauce and toss it in the pan and lower the heat.

6. Cook for another 5 minutes.

7. Once the tofu and the noodles are ready, combine them in a plate.

8. Add the fresh green onions on top.

NUTRITIONAL VALUE (per serving)

Fat: 26 g

Carbs: 58 g

Protein: 24 g

Total Calories: 485 Calories

Dinner

Eat Out Using the Vegan Guide Guidelines

Snacks

Coconut Chia Pudding

INGREDIENTS (4 Servings)

- 1 Can of Coconut Milk

- 1/4 Cup of Chia Seeds

- 1 Tbsp of Maple Syrup

- 1 tsp of Vanilla Extract

- 1 Cup of Berries

DIRECTIONS

1. Combine all of the ingredients in a bowl except the berries. Stir well and then transfer the mixture to a sealed container.

2. Let the chia seed pudding sit in the refrigerator for

3 hours or overnight.

3. Once it is ready you can separate it into 4

servings and add a handful of berries on top.

NUTRITIONAL VALUE (per serving)

Fat: 25 g

Carbs: 14 g

Protein: 5 g

Total Calories: 299 Calories

DAY SIX

Breakfast

Tofu Scramble

Tofu Scrambles

INGREDIENTS

- 4oz of Tofu

- 1/2 Cup of Red Bell Pepper

- 1 Cup of Spinach

- 1/4 Cup of Red Onion

- 1 Tbsp of Coconut Aminos

- 1 tsp of Coconut Oil

- 1 tsp of Turmeric

- 1/2 tsp of Sea Salt

- Pinch of Black Pepper

DIRECTIONS

1. Place a pan on medium heat and add the onions and peppers with the coconut oil.

2. Once the vegetables become translucent add the tofu to the pan and roughly break it down with a spatula.

3. Next add the coconut aminos, turmeric, salt and pepper and cook for another 5 minutes.

4. Add the spinach in the last 2 minutes to avoid wilting too much.

5. Enjoy!

NUTRITIONAL VALUE

Fat: 14 g

Carbs: 12 g

Protein: 15 g

Total Calories: 173 Calories

Lunch

Rainbow Salad

INGREDIENTS

- 1 Cup of Spinach

- 1/2 Zucchini (Preferably Spiralized)

- 1/2 Cup of Shredded Carrots

- 1/2 Cup of Shredded Red Cabbage

- Dressing:

- 1/2 Avocado

- 2 Tbsp of Extra Virgin Olive Oil

- Juice of 1/2 Lime

DIRECTIONS

1. Prepare all of the vegetables as listed above. I highly recommend creating different textures with your vegetables to add variety.

2. Place the mixed greens at the bottom of the bowl

then add all of the vegetables on top. Combine the avocado, extra virgin olive oil and the lime juice with salt and pepper to create a creamy dressing.

3. Serve with the dressing drizzled on top.

NUTRITIONAL VALUE

Fat: 42 g

Carbs: 23 g

Protein: 3 g

Total Calories: 457 Calories

Dinner

Sweet Potato Chickpea Curry

INGREDIENTS (2 Servings)

- 1.5 Cup (1 Small) of Sweet Potato

- 1 Can of Chickpeas

- 1 Cup of Coconut Milk

- 1/4 Cup of Onion

- 1 Can of Chopped Tomato

- 1 Tbsp of Olive Oil

- 1 Tbsp of Ground Turmeric

- 1 Tbsp of Ground Cumin

- 1 Tbsp of Ground Ginger

- 1 tsp of Sea Salt

DIRECTIONS

1. In a large pot heat the olive oil and the onions and the spices. Cook until the onions become translucent.

2. Next add in the rest of the ingredients, making sure that the sweet potatoes are completely covered with the liquid.

3. Bring the curry to a boil and then turn down to a simmer for about 40 minutes or until the sweet potatoes are completely done.

NUTRITIONAL VALUE (per serving)

Fat: 26 g

Carbs: 56 g

Protein: 13 g

Total Calories: 518 Calories

Snacks

Apple Pie Bites

INGREDIENTS (10 balls)

- 8 Medjool Dates

- 1 Cup of Dried Apples

- 1 Cup of Walnuts

- 1 tsp of Cinnamon

DIRECTIONS

1. Remove the pit from the dates. Combine all the ingredients in a food processor and mix until it forms a doughy mixture.

2. Form 10 balls with the mixture.

NUTRITIONAL VALUE (2 Balls)

Fat: 16 g

Carbs: 44 g

Protein: 5 g

Total Calories: 314 Calories

DAY SEVEN

Breakfast

Banana Pancakes

INGREDIENTS

- 1 Cup of Gluten Free Oatmeal

- 1/4 Cup of Almond Milk

- 1 Banana

- 1 Tbsp of Coconut Oil

- 2 tsp of Baking Powder

- 1/2 tsp of Cinnamon

DIRECTIONS

1. In a bowl combine all of the ingredients except for the coconut oil. Use a hand blender or a fork to mix everything together. Aim for a consistency similar to pancake batter.

2. Place a pan on medium heat and melt the coconut

oil. Slowly add the batter in the pan forming 5 inch diameter pancakes. Place the cover on and cook for a couple minutes on each side.

3. Repeat until you have cooked the whole batch. Be creative with your toppings, add any of your favourite clean foods. These may include but are not limited to berries, almond butter, coconut flakes and chopped nuts.

NUTRITIONAL VALUE

Fat: 24 g

Carbs: 30 g

Protein: 14 g

Total Calories: 378 Calories

Lunch

Sweet Potato Chickpea Curry (leftovers)

INGREDIENTS (2 Servings)

- 1.5 Cup (1 Small) of Sweet Potato

- 1 Can of Chickpeas

- 1 Cup of Coconut Milk

- 1/4 Cup of Onion

- 1 Can of Chopped Tomato

- 1 Tbsp of Olive Oil

- 1 Tbsp of Ground Turmeric

- 1 Tbsp of Ground Cumin

- 1 Tbsp of Ground Ginger

- 1 tsp of Sea Salt

DIRECTIONS

1. In a large pot heat the olive oil and the onions and the spices. Cook until the onions become translucent.

2. Next add in the rest of the ingredients, making sure that the sweet potatoes are completely covered with the liquid.

3. Bring the curry to a boil and then turn down to a simmer for about 40 minutes or until the sweet potatoes are completely done.

NUTRITIONAL VALUE (per serving)

Fat: 26 g

Carbs: 56 g

Protein: 13 g

Total Calories: 518 Calories

Dinner

Mexican Stuffed Peppers

INGREDIENTS (2 Servings)

- 2 Red Bell Peppers

- 1/4 Cup of Quinoa

- 1/2 Cup of Black Beans

- 1/2 Cup of Salsa

- 1/4 Cup of Fresh Chopped

- Cilantro

- 1 tsp of Paprika

- 1 tsp of Chili Powder

- Pinch of Sea Salt & Pepper

DIRECTIONS

1. Pre-heat the oven to 350F/175C and bake the peppers for 10 minutes on a baking tray.

2. Meanwhile cook the quinoa according to the directions on the packaging.

3. Mix all of the ingredients into a bowl then take the red pepper out of the oven and stuff them with the mixture.

4. Place the stuffed peppers back on the baking sheet and bake for another 10 minutes.

NUTRITIONAL VALUE (per serving)

Fat: 2 g

Carbs: 44 g

Protein: 12 g

Total Calories: 238 Calories

Snacks

Coconut Chia Pudding

INGREDIENTS (4 Servings)

- 1 Can of Coconut Milk

- 1/4 Cup of Chia Seeds

- 1 Tbsp of Maple Syrup

- 1 tsp of Vanilla Extract

- 1 Cup of Berries

DIRECTIONS

1. Combine all of the ingredients in a bowl except the berries. Stir well and then transfer the mixture to a sealed container.

2. Let the chia seed pudding sit in the refrigerator for

3 hours or overnight.

3. Once it is ready you can separate it into 4 servings and add a handful of berries on top.

NUTRITIONAL VALUE (per serving)

Fat: 25 g

Carbs: 14 g

Protein: 5 g

Total Calories: 299 Calories

WEEK FOUR

DAY ONE

Breakfast

Blueberry Smoothie

INGREDIENTS

- 1 Cup of Blueberries

- 1 Banana

- 1 Cup of Coconut Milk

- 1 Serving of Vanilla Protein Powder

- Handful of Ice

DIRECTIONS

1. Start by pouring the coconut milk into the blender to avoid the ingredients sticking at the bottom of the blender.

2. Next, throw in the blueberries, banana, collagen powder and the ice. Turn the blender on, starting at a low speed and increase as needed.

3. Once the liquid looks even, pour into a cup and enjoy immediately to conserve as many nutrients as possible.

NUTRITIONAL VALUE

Fat: 18 g

Carbs: 53 g

Protein: 20 g

Total Calories: 436 Calories

Lunch

Mexican Stuffed Peppers (leftovers)

INGREDIENTS (2 Servings)

- 2 Red Bell Peppers

- 1/4 Cup of Quinoa

- 1/2 Cup of Black Beans

- 1/2 Cup of Salsa

- 1/4 Cup of Fresh Chopped

- Cilantro

- 1 tsp of Paprika

- 1 tsp of Chili Powder

- Pinch of Sea Salt & Pepper

DIRECTIONS

1. Pre-heat the oven to 350F/175C and bake the peppers for 10 minutes on a baking tray.

2. Meanwhile cook the quinoa according to the directions on the packaging.

3. Mix all of the ingredients into a bowl then take the red pepper out of the oven and stuff them with the mixture.

4. Place the stuffed peppers back on the baking sheet and bake for another 10 minutes.

NUTRITIONAL VALUE (per serving)

Fat: 2 g

Carbs: 44 g

Protein: 12 g

Total Calories: 238 Calories

Dinner

Creamy Avocado Pasta

INGREDIENTS (2 Servings)

- 4 oz of Brown Rice Linguini

- 1 Avocado

- 1/2 Cup of Fresh Basil

- 2 Tbsp of Extra Virgin Olive Oil

- 2 Cloves of Garlic

- 1 Tbsp of Lemon Juice

- Pinch of Sea Salt and Pepper

DIRECTIONS

1. Start by preparing the pasta according to the directions on the packaging.

2. While the pasta is cooking start preparing the avocado cream sauce by combining all of the ingredients in a food processor.

3. Process until the consistency is nice and smooth.

4. Add the avocado cream sauce with the noodles once they are ready.

5. Feel free to add to favourite vegetarian protein source to this dish if you prefer a meal with higher protein.

NUTRITIONAL VALUE (per serving)

Fat: 27 g

Carbs: 47 g

Protein: 7 g

Total Calories: 446 Calories

Snacks

Oatmeal Cookies

INGREDIENTS (8 Cookies)

- 1 Cup of Gluten Free Oatmeal

- 1 Ripe Banana

- 1 tsp of Cinnamon

Optional: Add nuts, dried fruit or chocolate chips to customize the cookies to your liking.

DIRECTIONS

1. Preheat the oven at 375F/200C.

2. In a bowl, mash the banana and add the oats, cinnamon and any additional ingredients if you choose.

3. Combine until it forms a sticky and even mixture.

4. Divide the mixture in 8 equal cookies and place them on a baking sheet. Bake for 8 minutes.

NUTRITIONAL VALUE (per cookie)

Fat: 1 g

Carbs: 19 g

Protein: 3 g

Total Calories: 99 Calories

DAY TWO

Breakfast

Apple Cinnamon Cereal

INGREDIENTS

- 1 Apple

- 1/4 Cup of Coconut Chips

- 1/2 Cup of Almond Milk

- 2 Tbsp of Walnuts

- 2 Tbsp of Almonds

- 1/2 tsp of Ground Cinnamon

DIRECTIONS

1. Start by washing an apple and then cut it into small pieces.

2. Next combine the apple pieces and all the remaining ingredients into a small bowl.

3. Add any other nuts and seeds that you enjoy to add texture to this grain free cereal.

NUTRITIONAL VALUE

Fat: 28 g

Carbs: 19 g

Protein: 8 g

Total Calories: 350 Calories

Lunch

Creamy Avocado Pasta (leftovers)

INGREDIENTS (2 Servings)

- 4 oz of Brown Rice Linguini

- 1 Avocado

- 1/2 Cup of Fresh Basil

- 2 Tbsp of Extra Virgin Olive Oil

- 2 Cloves of Garlic

- 1 Tbsp of Lemon Juice

- Pinch of Sea Salt and Pepper

DIRECTIONS

1. Start by preparing the pasta according to the directions on the packaging.

2. While the pasta is cooking start preparing the avocado cream sauce by combining all of the ingredients in a food processor.

3. Process until the consistency is nice and smooth.

4. Add the avocado cream sauce with the noodles once they are ready.

5. Feel free to add to favourite vegetarian protein source to this dish if you prefer a meal with higher protein.

NUTRITIONAL VALUE (per serving)

Fat: 27 g

Carbs: 47 g

Protein: 7 g

Total Calories: 446 Calories

Dinner

Falafel Salad

INGREDIENTS (2 Servings)

- 1 Can of Chickpeas

- 1/4 Cup of Red Onion

- 1/2 Cup of Fresh Parsley

- 1 Cloves of Garlic

- 1/2 tsp of Cumin

- Pinch of Sea Salt & Pepper

- 2 Cup of Fresh Greens

- 2 Tbsp of Tahini

- 1 tsp of Lemon Juice

DIRECTIONS

1. Pre-heat the oven to 400F.

2. Combine the chickpeas, red onions, garlic, cumin, parsley and cilantro in a food processor.

Process for a few seconds, leaving the mixture a little bit chunky.

3. Form 8 small patties with the mixture and then refrigerate for an hour to let them set.

4. Bake for 45 minutes, flipping them half way.

5. While the falafel are baking prepare the salad and the dressing by combining the tahini and lemon juice.

NUTRITIONAL VALUE (4 Falafel)

Fat: 3 g

Carbs: 29 g

Protein: 9 g

Total Calories: 171 Calories

Snacks

Easy Trail Mix

INGREDIENTS (3 servings)

- 1/2 Cup of Coconut Chips

- 1/4 Cup of Almonds

- 1/4 Cup of Pumpkin Seeds

DIRECTIONS

1. Place all of the ingredients in an air tight jar and store somewhere cool or immediately divide the trail mix into 3 portions.

NUTRITIONAL VALUE (per serving)

Fat: 20 g

Carbs: 9 g

Protein: 10 g

Total Calories: 256 Calories

DAY THREE

Breakfast

Blueberry Smoothie

INGREDIENTS

- 1 Cup of Blueberries

- 1 Banana

- 1 Cup of Coconut Milk

- 1 Serving of Vanilla Protein Powder

- Handful of Ice

DIRECTIONS

1. Start by pouring the coconut milk into the blender to avoid the ingredients sticking at the bottom of the blender.

2. Next, throw in the blueberries, banana, collagen powder and the ice. Turn the blender on, starting at a low speed and increase as needed.

3. Once the liquid looks even, pour into a cup and

enjoy immediately to conserve as many nutrients as possible.

NUTRITIONAL VALUE

Fat: 18 g

Carbs: 53 g

Protein: 20 g

Total Calories: 436 Calories

Lunch

Falafel Salad (leftovers)

INGREDIENTS (2 Servings)

- 1 Can of Chickpeas

- 1/4 Cup of Red Onion

- 1/2 Cup of Fresh Parsley

- 1 Cloves of Garlic

- 1/2 tsp of Cumin

- Pinch of Sea Salt & Pepper

- 2 Cup of Fresh Greens

- 2 Tbsp of Tahini

- 1 tsp of Lemon Juice

DIRECTIONS

1. Pre-heat the oven to 400F.

2. Combine the chickpeas, red onions, garlic, cumin, parsley and cilantro in a food processor.

Process for a few seconds, leaving the mixture a little bit chunky.

3. Form 8 small patties with the mixture and then refrigerate for an hour to let them set.

4. Bake for 45 minutes, flipping them half way.

5. While the falafel are baking prepare the salad and the dressing by combining the tahini and lemon juice.

NUTRITIONAL VALUE (4 Falafel)

Fat: 3 g

Carbs: 29 g

Protein: 9 g

Total Calories: 171 Calories

Dinner

Tofu Almond Butter Stir Fry

INGREDIENTS (2 Servings)

- 8 oz of Tofu

- 2 Cups of Broccoli

- 1 Red Bell Pepper

- 4 Mushrooms

- 1/4 Cup of Red Onion

- 2 Tbsp of Coconut Oil

- Almond Butter Sauce:

- 1/4 Cup of Coconut Aminos

- 2 Tbsp of Almond Butter

DIRECTIONS

1. Chop all the vegetables in bite size pieces.

2. In a large pan place the coconut oil and the tofu cubed on medium heat and cook for a few minutes.

3. Once the tofu has begun to brown a little bit add all of the chopped vegetables and the sauce and cook for another 5-10 minutes (depending on how you like your vegetables).

4. Turn the heat off, take the cover off and let the sauce thicken up for a few minutes before serving.

NUTRITIONAL VALUE (per serving)

Fat: 43 g

Carbs: 49 g

Protein: 25 g

Total Calories: 563 Calories

Snacks

Oatmeal Cookies

INGREDIENTS (8 Cookies)

- 1 Cup of Gluten Free Oatmeal

- 1 Ripe Banana

- 1 tsp of Cinnamon

Optional: Add nuts, dried fruit or chocolate chips to

customize the cookies to your liking.

DIRECTIONS

1. Preheat the oven at 375F/200C.

2. In a bowl, mash the banana and add the oats, cinnamon and any additional ingredients if you choose.

3. Combine until it forms a sticky and even mixture.

4. Divide the mixture in 8 equal cookies and place them on a baking sheet. Bake for 8 minutes.

NUTRITIONAL VALUE (per cookie)

Fat: 1 g

Carbs: 19 g

Protein: 3 g

Total Calories: 99 Calories

DAY FOUR

Breakfast

Apple Cinnamon Cereal

INGREDIENTS

- 1 Apple

- 1/4 Cup of Coconut Chips

- 1/2 Cup of Almond Milk

- 2 Tbsp of Walnuts

- 2 Tbsp of Almonds

- 1/2 tsp of Ground Cinnamon

DIRECTIONS

1. Start by washing an apple and then cut it into small pieces.

2. Next combine the apple pieces and all the remaining ingredients into a small bowl.

3. Add any other nuts and seeds that you enjoy to add texture to this grain free cereal.

NUTRITIONAL VALUE

Fat: 28 g

Carbs: 19 g

Protein: 8 g

Total Calories: 350 Calories

Lunch

Tofu Almond Butter Stir Fry (leftovers)

INGREDIENTS (2 Servings)

- 8 oz of Tofu

- 2 Cups of Broccoli

- 1 Red Bell Pepper

- 4 Mushrooms

- 1/4 Cup of Red Onion

- 2 Tbsp of Coconut Oil

- Almond Butter Sauce:

- 1/4 Cup of Coconut Aminos

- 2 Tbsp of Almond Butter

DIRECTIONS

1. Chop all the vegetables in bite size pieces.

2. In a large pan place the coconut oil and the tofu cubed on medium heat and cook for a few minutes.

3. Once the tofu has begun to brown a little bit add all of the chopped vegetables and the sauce and cook for another 5-10 minutes (depending on how you like your vegetables).

4. Turn the heat off, take the cover off and let the sauce thicken up for a few minutes before serving.

NUTRITIONAL VALUE (per serving)

Fat: 43 g

Carbs: 49 g

Protein: 25 g

Total Calories: 563 Calories

Dinner

Black Bean Burgers

INGREDIENTS (2 Servings)

- 1 Can of Black Beans

- 1/4 Cup of Gluten Free Oatmeal

- 1/4 Cup of Chopped Onion

- 2 Cloves of Garlic

- 1/4 Cup of Fresh Parsley

- 1 tsp of Chilli

- 1/2 tsp of Cayenne Powder

- 1/2 tsp of Sea Salt

- 1/2 tsp of Pepper

DIRECTIONS

1. Drain and rinse the black beans and pat dry with paper towel.

2. Place all of the ingredients in a food processor and the mixture becomes sticky.

3. Form 4 patties and cook on the stove top on medium heat with coconut oil.

4. Fry the patty for about 3-5 minutes each side and then you can add any of your favourite toppings to the burger patties.

NUTRITIONAL VALUE (2 Patties)

Fat: 2 g

Carbs: 46 g

Protein: 16 g

Total Calories: 262 Calories

Snacks

Easy Trail Mix

INGREDIENTS (3 servings)

- 1/2 Cup of Coconut Chips

- 1/4 Cup of Almonds

- 1/4 Cup of Pumpkin Seeds

DIRECTIONS

1. Place all of the ingredients in an air tight jar and store somewhere cool or immediately divide the trail mix into 3 portions.

NUTRITIONAL VALUE (per serving)

Fat: 20 g

Carbs: 9 g

Protein: 10 g

Total Calories: 256 Calories

DAY FIVE

Breakfast

Blueberry Smoothie

INGREDIENTS

- 1 Cup of Blueberries

- 1 Banana

- 1 Cup of Coconut Milk

- 1 Serving of Vanilla Protein Powder

- Handful of Ice

DIRECTIONS

1. Start by pouring the coconut milk into the blender to avoid the ingredients sticking at the bottom of the blender.

2. Next, throw in the blueberries, banana, collagen powder and the ice. Turn the blender on, starting at a low speed and increase as needed.

3. Once the liquid looks even, pour into a cup and enjoy immediately to conserve as many nutrients as

possible.

NUTRITIONAL VALUE

Fat: 18 g

Carbs: 53 g

Protein: 20 g

Total Calories: 436 Calories

Lunch

Black Bean Burgers (leftovers)

INGREDIENTS (2 Servings)

- 1 Can of Black Beans

- 1/4 Cup of Gluten Free Oatmeal

- 1/4 Cup of Chopped Onion

- 2 Cloves of Garlic

- 1/4 Cup of Fresh Parsley

- 1 tsp of Chilli

- 1/2 tsp of Cayenne Powder

- 1/2 tsp of Sea Salt

- 1/2 tsp of Pepper

DIRECTIONS

1. Drain and rinse the black beans and pat dry with paper towel.

2. Place all of the ingredients in a food processor and the mixture becomes sticky.

3. Form 4 patties and cook on the stove top on medium heat with coconut oil.

4. Fry the patty for about 3-5 minutes each side and then you can add any of your favourite toppings to the burger patties.

NUTRITIONAL VALUE (2 Patties)

Fat: 2 g

Carbs: 46 g

Protein: 16 g

Total Calories: 262 Calories

Dinner

Eat Out Using the Vegan Guide

Guidelines

Snacks

Oatmeal Cookies

INGREDIENTS (8 Cookies)

- 1 Cup of Gluten Free Oatmeal

- 1 Ripe Banana

- 1 tsp of Cinnamon

Optional: Add nuts, dried fruit or chocolate chips to customize the cookies to your liking.

DIRECTIONS

1. Preheat the oven at 375F/200C.

2. In a bowl, mash the banana and add the oats, cinnamon and any additional ingredients if you choose.

3. Combine until it forms a sticky and even mixture.

4. Divide the mixture in 8 equal cookies and place them on a baking sheet. Bake for 8 minutes.

NUTRITIONAL VALUE (per cookie)

Fat: 1 g

Carbs: 19 g

Protein: 3 g

Total Calories: 99 Calories

DAY SIX

Breakfast

Apple Cinnamon Cereal

INGREDIENTS

- 1 Apple

- 1/4 Cup of Coconut Chips

- 1/2 Cup of Almond Milk

- 2 Tbsp of Walnuts

- 2 Tbsp of Almonds

- 1/2 tsp of Ground Cinnamon

DIRECTIONS

1. Start by washing an apple and then cut it into small pieces.

2. Next combine the apple pieces and all the remaining ingredients into a small bowl.

3. Add any other nuts and seeds that you enjoy to add texture to this grain free cereal.

NUTRITIONAL VALUE

Fat: 28 g

Carbs: 19 g

Protein: 8 g

Total Calories: 350 Calories

Lunch

Crunchy Kale Salad

INGREDIENTS

- 2 Cups of Kale

- 1 Carrot

- 1/2 Avocado

- 1/2 Cup of Chickpeas

- Dressing:

- 1 Tbsp of Tahini

- 1 Tbsp of Lemon Juice

DIRECTIONS

1. Preheat the oven to 350F/175C.

2. Drain and rinse the chickpeas. Dry them with a paper towel and spread them evenly on a baking tray. Bake for 45 minutes.

3. Meanwhile prepare the vegetables by rinsing and chopping up the kale, peeling and shredding the carrots and cutting the avocado into small cubes. Set the vegetables aside.

4. Combine all the dressing ingredients into a bowl and whisk together until it forms a smooth consistency.

5. Place all of the vegetables to a bowl with the baked chickpeas and then drizzle the dressing on top.

NUTRITIONAL VALUE

Fat: 22 g

Carbs: 40 g

Protein: 16 g

Total Calories: 431 Calories

Dinner

Zoodles & Lentil Meatballs

INGREDIENTS (2 Servings)

- 2 Zucchinis

- 1 Cup of Cooked Lentils

- 1/4 Cup of Quinoa

- 1/2 Cup of Almond Flour

- 1/4 Cup of Chopped Onion

- 2 Garlic Cloves

- 2 Tbsp of Italian Seasoning

- 400 ml of Marinara Sauce

DIRECTIONS

1. Start by preparing the lentils and quinoa according to directions on the package.

2. Once the lentils and quinoa are ready add everything except for the marinara sauce and zucchini in the food processor.

3. Process until it is completely smooth. Roll out 10 small "meatballs" with the lentil mixture.

4. Heat olive oil in a large pan and cook the meatballs for 5 minutes.

5. Next add the marinara sauce to the pan, mix in with the meatballs and cook for another 5 minutes.

6. Serve over spiralized zucchini. If you do not have a spiralizer you can create linguini noodles out of zucchini with a regular peeler.

NUTRITIONAL VALUE (per serving)

Fat: 18 g

Carbs: 55 g

Protein: 20 g

Total Calories: 441 Calories

Snacks

Easy Trail Mix

INGREDIENTS (3 servings)

- 1/2 Cup of Coconut Chips

- 1/4 Cup of Almonds

- 1/4 Cup of Pumpkin Seeds

DIRECTIONS

1. Place all of the ingredients in an air tight jar and store somewhere cool or immediately divide the trail mix into 3 portions.

NUTRITIONAL VALUE (per serving)

Fat: 20 g

Carbs: 9 g

Protein: 10 g

Total Calories: 256 Calories

DAY SEVEN

Breakfast

Banana Pancakes

INGREDIENTS

- 1 Cup of Gluten Free Oatmeal

- 1/4 Cup of Almond Milk

- 1 Banana

- 1 Tbsp of Coconut Oil

- 2 tsp of Baking Powder

- 1/2 tsp of Cinnamon

DIRECTIONS

1. In a bowl combine all of the ingredients except for the coconut oil. Use a hand blender or a fork to mix everything together. Aim for a consistency similar to pancake batter.

2. Place a pan on medium heat and melt the coconut oil. Slowly add the batter in the pan forming 5 inch diameter pancakes. Place the cover on and cook for a couple minutes on each side.

3. Repeat until you have cooked the whole batch. Be creative with your toppings, add any of your favourite clean foods. These may include but are not limited to berries, almond butter, coconut flakes

and chopped nuts.

NUTRITIONAL VALUE

Fat: 24 g

Carbs: 30 g

Protein: 14 g

Total Calories: 378 Calories

Lunch

Zoodles & Lentil Meatballs (leftovers)

INGREDIENTS (2 Servings)

- 2 Zucchinis

- 1 Cup of Cooked Lentils

- 1/4 Cup of Quinoa

- 1/2 Cup of Almond Flour

- 1/4 Cup of Chopped Onion

- 2 Garlic Cloves

- 2 Tbsp of Italian Seasoning

- 400 ml of Marinara Sauce

DIRECTIONS

1. Start by preparing the lentils and quinoa according to directions on the package.

2. Once the lentils and quinoa are ready add everything except for the marinara sauce and zucchini in the food processor.

3. Process until it is completely smooth. Roll out 10 small "meatballs" with the lentil mixture.

4. Heat olive oil in a large pan and cook the meatballs for 5 minutes.

5. Next add the marinara sauce to the pan, mix in with the meatballs and cook for another 5 minutes.

6. Serve over spiralized zucchini. If you do not have a spiralizer you can create linguini noodles out of zucchini with a regular peeler.

NUTRITIONAL VALUE (per serving)

Fat: 18 g

Carbs: 55 g

Protein: 20 g

Total Calories: 441 Calories

Dinner

Quinoa Tabouleh

INGREDIENTS

- 1/4 Cup of Quinoa

- 1/2 Cup of Fresh Parsley

- 2 Tomatoes

- 2 Tbsp of Pine Nuts

- 1 Tbsp of Tahini

- 1 Tbsp of Olive Oil

- Juice of 1/2 Lemon

DIRECTIONS

1. Start by preparing the quinoa according to the directions on the packaging.

2. While the quinoa is cooking start chopping the parsley and the tomatoes.

3. Once the quinoa is done let it cool down for a

little bit and then add all of the remaining ingredients.

4. Mix well and serve cold.

NUTRITIONAL VALUE

Fat: 29 g

Carbs: 36 g

Protein: 10 g

Total Calories: 423 Calories

Snacks

Oatmeal Cookies

INGREDIENTS (8 Cookies)

- 1 Cup of Gluten Free Oatmeal

- 1 Ripe Banana

- 1 tsp of Cinnamon

Optional: Add nuts, dried fruit or chocolate chips to customize the cookies to your liking.

DIRECTIONS

1. Preheat the oven at 375F/200C.

2. In a bowl, mash the banana and add the oats, cinnamon and any additional ingredients if you choose.

3. Combine until it forms a sticky and even mixture.

4. Divide the mixture in 8 equal cookies and place them on a baking sheet. Bake for 8 minutes.

NUTRITIONAL VALUE (per cookie)

Fat: 1 g

Carbs: 19 g

Protein: 3 g

Total Calories: 99 Calories

CHAPTER EIGHT

GROCERY SHOPPING TIPS AND LIST

1. Ingredients like coconut oil and olive oil are only on the first week's grocery list because they are used daily so be aware if you run out you will need to re-purchase these.

2. Ingredients like Almond Butter, Coconut Aminos, Tahini, Almond Flour, Chia Seeds, Oats, Quinoa, and baking ingredients are listed in the grocery lists usually as a few tablespoons but I highly recommend to buy these in bulk and before heading to the grocery store check if you already have them in your pantry.

3. The vegetables are sometimes rounded off, for example when you need two cups of broccoli in a recipe you will only be able to purchase a full head. In this case I encourage you to use the extra vegetables in other meals or use it as dipping vegetables if hummus is your planned snack for the week.

4. There are also recipes with protein powder as an ingredient. Protein powders can be bought by the serving or in a big container. I recommend going to the container if it is something you plan on using past the 28 Day Meal Plan. If not then finding single servings may be best.

5. Bananas! There are always bananas needed in smoothies every week so if you buy too many or they are on sale feel free to stock up and freeze them.

6. Many of these recipes call for fresh herbs like parsley and basil. To save money I recommend getting these two herbs as a small plant. They are very easy to maintain and don't cost much.

7. Use any excess vegetables to snack on during the week when you are hungry.

8. Lastly, always check the fridge and pantry before you head out to the grocery store with your list to make sure there are no left overs.

GROCERY LIST - WEEK 1

Fruits & Vegetables

3 Bananas

1/2 Cup of Berries

1 Lemon

1 Lime

4 Avocados

1/2 Cup of Guacamole

4 Cups of Arugula

4 Cups of Spinach

2 Cups Kale

1/4 Cup of Fresh Chopped Cilantro

2 Sweet Potatoes

4 Red Bell Peppers

1/2 Zucchini

1 Carrot

1 Small Head of Red Cabbage

2 Tomatoes

1 Cucumber

1 Stalks of Celery

2 Portobello Mushroom

1 Cup of Bean Sprouts

1/2 Cup of Green Onions

1 Red Onion

1 Onion

4 Cloves of Garlic

Grains, Beans & Legumes

4 oz of Brown Rice Noodles

1 Brown Rice Tortilla Wrap

1/2 Cup of Brown Rice

1/4 Cup of Quinoa

2 1/2 Cup of Gluten Free Oatmeal

1 Can + 1/2 Cup of Black Bean

2 Cans + 2 Cups of Chickpeas

Nuts & Seeds

1 1/4 Cup of Almonds

3 Tbsp of Chia Seeds

Baking Supplies

Baking Powder

1/2 Cup of Shredded Coconut

2 Tbsp of Raw Cacao Powder

8 Medjool Dates

Condiments

Organic Coconut Oil

Extra Virgin Olive Oil

Balsamic Vinegar

1 Can of Chopped Tomato

1/2 Cup of Salsa

6 1/4 Cups of Almond Milk

1 Cup of Coconut Milk

1/4 Cup of Coconut Aminos

1/4 Cup + 2 Tbsp of Tahini

2 Tbsp of Vegan Mayo

2 Tbsp of Almond Butter

Herbs & Spices

Paprika

Garlic Powder

Onion Powder

Cayenne Powder

Ground Turmeric

Ground Cumin

Ground Ginger

Chilli Powder

Ground Cinnamon

Extra

8 oz of Tofu

3 Servings of Vanilla Protein Powder

GROCERY LIST - WEEK 2

Fruits & Vegetables

3 Bananas

3 Cups of Raspberries

2 Avocados

1 Lemon

1 Lime

2 Cups of Kale

2 Cup of Fresh Greens

1 1/4 Cup of Fresh Parsley

1/2 Cup of Fresh Basil

1 Small Head of Broccoli

2 Zucchinis

1 Red Bell Pepper

7 Carrots

2 Tomatoes

1/2 Cup of Cherry Tomatoes

1 Small Cucumber

4 Mushrooms

1 Red Onion

1 Onion

7 Cloves of Garlic

Grains, Beans & Legumes

4 oz of Brown Rice Linguini

1/2 Cup of Quinoa

2 3/4 Cup of Gluten Free Oatmeal

1 Can + 1/2 Cup of Chickpeas

1 Can of Black Beans

1 Cup of Cooked Lentils

Nuts & Seeds

1/2 Cup + 2 Tbsp of Chia Seeds

1/4 Cups of Sesame Seeds

1/4 Cups of Sunflower Seeds

2 Tbsp of Pine Nuts

Baking Supplies

1/2 Cup of Almond Flour

3 Tbsp of Raw Cacao Powder

3 Tbsp of Maple Syrup

Condiments

400 ml of Marinara Sauce

3 Cups of Coconut Milk

3 1/4 Cups of Almond Milk

1/4 Cup of Coconut Aminos

1/4 Cup + 1 Tbsp of Almond Butter

1/4 Cup of Tahini

Herbs & Spices

Italian Seasoning

Herb Mix Seasoning

Extra

8 oz of Tofu

3 Servings of Vanilla Protein Powder

3 Servings of Chocolate Protein Powder

GROCERY LIST - WEEK 3

Fruits & Vegetables

4 Bananas

1 Cup of Berries

1 Lemon

1 Lime

4 Avocados

1/2 Cup of Guacamole

4 Cups of Arugula

2 Cups Kale

2 Cups of Spinach

1/4 Cup of Fresh Chopped Cilantro

2 Sweet Potatoes

4 1/2 Red Bell Peppers

1/2 Zucchini

1 Carrot

1 Small Head of Red Cabbage

2 Tomatoes

1 Small Cucumber

1 Stalks of Celery

2 Portobello Mushroom

1 Cup of Bean Sprouts

1/2 Cup of Green Onions

1 Red Onion

1 Onion

3 Cloves of Garlic

Grains, Beans & Legumes

4 oz of Brown Rice Noodles

1 Brown Rice Tortilla Wrap

1/2 Cup of Brown Rice

1/4 Cup of Quinoa

1 Cups of Gluten Free Oatmeal

1 Can + 1/2 Cup of Black Bean

1 Can + 2 Cups of Chickpeas

Nuts & Seeds

1 Cup of Walnuts

1/4 Cup of Chia Seeds

Baking Supplies

1 Cup of Apple Chips

 1/4 Cup + 2 Tbsp of Raw Cacao Powder

1 Tbsp of Maple Syrup

1 tsp of Vanilla Extract

8 Medjool Dates

Condiments

1 Can of Chopped Tomato

1/2 Cup of Salsa

3 1/4 Cups of Almond Milk

1 Can + 1 Cup of Coconut Milk

1/4 Cup + 1 Tbsp of Coconut Aminos

2 Tbsp of Vegan Mayo

2 Tbsp of Tahini

2 Tbsp of Almond Butter

Extra

12 oz of Tofu

3 Servings of Chocolate Protein Powder

GROCERY LIST - WEEK 4

Fruits & Vegetables

4 Bananas

3 Apples

3 Cups of Blueberries

2 Avocados

1 Lemon

2 Cups of Kale

2 Cup of Fresh Greens

1 1/4 Cup of Fresh Parsley

1/2 Cup of Fresh Basil

1 Small Head of Broccoli

2 Zucchinis

1 Red Bell Pepper

1 Carrot

2 Tomatoes

1/2 Cup of Cherry Tomatoes

1 Small Cucumber

4 Mushrooms

1 Red Onion

1 Onion

7 Cloves of Garlic

Grains, Beans & Legumes

4 oz of Brown Rice Linguini

1/2 Cup of Quinoa

1 1/4 Cup of Gluten Free Oatmeal

1 Can + 1/2 Cup of Chickpeas

1 Can of Black Beans

1 Cup of Cooked Lentils

Nuts & Seeds

1/2 + 2 Tbsp of Almonds

1/4 Cup + 2 Tbsp of Walnuts

1/4 Cup of Pumpkin Seeds

2 Tbsp of Pine Nuts

Baking Supplies

1 1/4 Cup of Coconut Chips

1/2 Cup of Almond Flour

Condiments

400 ml of Marinara Sauce

3 Cups of Coconut Milk

1 1/2 Cup of Almond Milk

1/4 Cup of Coconut Aminos

1/4 Cup of Tahini

2 Tbsp of Almond Butter

Extra

8 oz of Tofu

3 Servings of Vanilla Protein Powder

CONCLUSION

Vegetables will be the basis for enhancing health. As a result of this, filling your daily diet using as lots of green leafy vegetables as well as various vegetables of different types ought to be your everyday aim. By ingesting an range of veggies, you're filling with foods that are unsalted which provide each the vitamins, minerals, minerals, and phytonutrients your body has to protect itself. Additionally, vegetables do not contain cholesterol, and also the soluble fiber they feature helps reduce the bad cholesterol in your system. Most are extremely low in carbs. All meats, such as fish would be the reverse; they feature cholesterol and don't contain fiber. The simple fact that all meat includes cholesterol, without a fiber, which results in the next step in attaining nutritional excellence. The next step would be to eliminate or radically decrease the sum of all sorts of meat from the diet. Research clearly indicates that people who have high amounts of legumes of all sorts have greater incidences of cardiovascular issues. The connection of beef intake to heart troubles also carries more than other animal products. This usually means there are unwanted side effects from ingestion of eggs and legumes too. The next step would be to substitute processed grains with whole grains. And lastly, read labels and prevent too many processed additives and substances in your meals as you can.

A frequent objection from the firehouse to modifications such as those mentioned previously is the perceived requirement for eggs, poultry, and milk for a source of nourishment and calcium. This emptiness is easily debunked from the advantages of a"complete foods, plant-based diet." there's more protein in veggies such as broccoli and romaine lettuce compared to beef. Furthermore, a well-rounded, plant-based diet can offer numerous sources of protein like legumes, brown rice, and kale. And like calcium, though milk is indeed a wealthy supply, various studies have proven that since it's delivered in the kind of animal protein, milk might really harm bone health by producing an acidic state within the entire body. Rich sources of salt can be found in leafy green veggies such as collard greens and greens in addition to fortified sources like almond milk and orange juice, which makes the requirement to eat milk nonexistent.

www.ingramcontent.com/pod-product-compliance
Lightning Source LLC
Chambersburg PA
CBHW031048250726

48655CB00004B/1353